MW00777727

THE COLD THERAPY CODE

REDISCOVER YOUR VITALITY THROUGH COLD
EXPOSURE - THE 3 SIMPLE CRYOTHERAPY METHODS
FOR REDUCING STRESS, IMPROVING SLEEP, AND
INCREASING ENERGY

JAMES H. SMART

WWW.JAMESHSMART.COM

Text Copyright © James H. Smart

The information contained in this book is not designed to replace or take the place of any form of medicine or professional medical advice. The information in this book has been provided for educational and entertainment purposes only.

The information contained in this book has been compiled from sources deemed reliable, and it is accurate to the best of the Author's knowledge; however, the Author cannot guarantee its accuracy and validity and cannot be held liable for any errors or omissions. Changes are periodically made to this book. You must consult your doctor or get professional medical advice before using any of the suggested remedies, techniques, or information in this book.

Upon using the information contained in this book, you agree to hold harmless the Author from and against any damages, costs, and expenses, including any legal fees potentially resulting from the application of any of the information provided by this guide. This disclaimer applies to any damages or injury caused by the use and application, whether directly or indirectly, of any advice or information presented, whether for breach of contract, tort, negligence, personal injury, criminal intent, or under any other cause of action.

You agree to accept all risks of using the information presented inside this book. You need to consult a professional medical practitioner in order to ensure you are able and healthy enough to participate in this program.

CONTENTS

JUST FOR YOU...

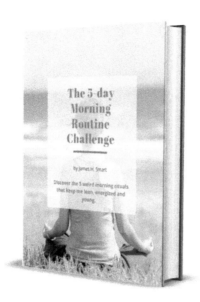

A FREE GIFT FOR OUR READERS

The 5-Day Morning Routine Challenge.
Discover the 5 weird morning rituals that keep me lean,
energized and young.
Start today by visiting the link:
www.jameshsmart.com

INTRODUCTION

It is estimated that around 1.5 billion people around the world live with chronic pain. Often, we ignore the early warning signs of pain, but that's not wise as it can lead to more serious problems down the road. People suffer from a variety of ailments that negatively affect their daily lives, including arthritis, headaches, abdominal pain, back pain, muscle soreness, anxiety, and depression. Suffering from these conditions is completely unnecessary because there may be a simple solution to ease or heal the ailment.

As we age, many of us feel that our health and vitality are slipping away and that we are powerless to stop the seemingly inevitable downward spiral. I was one of those people.

However, I am now a firm believer that it doesn't have to be that way, and I'm here to tell you that it doesn't have to be that way for you either. You can choose a different future. A future free from pain and struggle. A future where you feel invigorated and empowered every single day.

Is Cold Exposure the same as Cryotherapy?

The words are often used interchangeably, so I thought it would be a good idea to establish what they mean in the context of this book. Briefly, cryotherapy is any kind of therapy that uses ice or very cold (sometimes extremely cold) temperatures to treat part of your body or your whole body for any particular reason. The reasons we use cryotherapy and the benefits thereof are detailed throughout the book.

Cold exposure, on the other hand, is a relatively new term that refers to a type of cryotherapy that relies less on chambers and gadgets and more on cold showers, ice baths, swimming in icy cold lakes, and walking outside in freezing cold weather wearing nothing more than swimming trunks. Sound crazy? Bear with me. You're about to learn about the short- and long-term benefits of cold exposure and cryotherapy in a way that I hope will convince you to give it a try.

In essence, both cryotherapy and cold exposure expose your body to extremely cold temperatures for short periods of time. They both work at a cellular level to accelerate recovery. The extreme cold temperatures improve blood circulation, speeding up the removal of toxins. The oxygen and nutrient-rich blood flow also improves organ function while reducing inflammation. Most notably, the extreme cold stimulates skin sensors, causing the release of endorphins, the body's natural pain inhibitors and mood elevators.

Cold exposure has been a daily practice for professional sports teams and athletes like Lebron James, Cristiano Ronaldo, Allyson Felix, and Novak Djokovic for many years. Post-exercise cold exposure treatment sessions help sportspeople ease muscle tension, rapidly accelerating recovery, and decreasing the effect of delayed onset muscle soreness (DOMS). A-list celebrities like Tony Robbins, Will Smith, Lady Gaga, Jennifer Aniston, Kevin Hart, and countless others are also firm believers in the powerful benefits of cryotherapy.

You will probably be surprised to know that these celebrities also keep themselves looking youthful with the help of cryotherapy. Cryotherapy is a relatively low-cost wellness treatment that promises everything, from healing chronic sports injuries and improving your state of mind to reducing anxiety and prolonging your life. The great news is that you don't have to be rich and famous to benefit from it because cold exposure does the same at no cost. Cold exposure, also referred to as cold therapy, can help anybody, even those who don't have the budget to pay for cryotherapy sessions.

Despite cryotherapy being an ancient form of healing, I don't believe it has had the recognition it deserves. Because cold water is relatively inexpensive to access for most people, corporations have no financial incentive to promote it, unlike the big pharma companies that make billions every year from selling drugs.

No one exemplifies the cold therapy movement better than the Dutch guru Wim Hof, whose remarkable ability to regulate his body heat in the extreme cold has sparked intense scientific study and earned him the name "The Iceman." Thanks to Hof, scientists in the US and Europe are starting to better understand how cold adaptation might help combat autoimmune diseases and chronic pain.

Personally, cryotherapy has changed my life for the better. In my early 20s, I was a semi-professional athlete. As a sportsman, I always strived to improve my mental and physical performance. But, at the age of twenty-five, I suffered a severe eye injury and was forced to retire. The ophthalmologist told me that I would never be able to play the sport I loved again. That was a difficult message to comprehend. My whole identity was wrapped up in being a sportsman. To have that taken away prematurely was a bitter pill to swallow.

The few months following my retirement from sport were particularly difficult. I developed back pain, joint stiffness, anxiety, lethargy, and weight gain due to a lack of physical activity and poor eating habits. My health was spiraling out of control. Prescription medicines only temporarily masked my pain, my sleep patterns were erratic, and my energy levels and motivation were at an all-time low.

To improve my life, I had to take full responsibility for the bad shape that I was in. It was no one's fault but my own. The moment you take responsibility and stop believing that you are a victim of your circumstances, you realize that there is a way out. Owning your situation (however bad you may think it is) and knowing that you are bigger than any circumstance has enormous power.

No matter your current situation or your interest in cryotherapy, I will walk you through this book step-by-step, ensuring you get the right information to get the best results from cryotherapy. I am passionate about this subject, and I'm eager to spread the word about its amazing benefits. I want you to experience the profound benefits of cold exposure, just like I have. I went from being overweight, sick, and broke to lean, healthy, and wealthy. You, too, can transform your life. You are about to learn how cold therapy can reduce chronic pain, reduce stress, improve sleep, and increase your energy.

After the horrors of Covid-19, which has claimed the lives of millions of people globally, our health, wellness, and having a strong immune system have never been more important.

In this book, you will rediscover the true connection between your mind and body and learn about the science that allows us to push past our physical limitations. This book is about taking back control of your life and your health.

Important note

Cold exposure offers many health and wellness benefits, many of which are listed and expanded upon in this book. However, the cold is an element that needs to be treated with the utmost respect.

Cold showers are great and probably safe for most people to practice; extreme cold exposure is on a completely different level, though. When you start to include outdoor cold exposure with your cold therapy practice, I advise extreme caution.

As much as I want you to get the maximum benefit from cold therapy, I want you to *live* to advocate the benefits.

Always ...

... Seek medical advice first.

... Pay attention to your body.

... Be responsible.

1

THE SCIENCE OF COLD EXPOSURE

"If we always choose comfort, we never learn the deepest capabilities of our mind or body." — Wim "The Iceman" Hoff

---

I'm sure you've seen Sci-Fi movies where the villain has a chip implanted in their body or uses gene-editing technology to gain superpowers. All these methods are called biohacking. Biohacking is a word that unites the hi-tech, wellness, anti-aging, and science communities. At its most basic, it means doing things to your body or mind to make them function better.

Biohacking as a concept may be as simple as making small changes to your diet or lifestyle to optimize your body's overall performance. It can even be taken to extremes, such as using implant technology and genetic engineering. There are numerous biohacking methods out there, and this is an area of research that is constantly evolving.

Cryotherapy is one type of biohacking that aims to improve an individual's physical and mental well-being using extremely cold temperatures. It is a drug-free intervention with huge benefits, such as offering relief to those who suffer from certain ailments, allowing athletes to recover faster and, therefore, perform at their best, and even offering well-being through relaxation and stress relief. Despite the rise in awareness and popularity of cryotherapy in recent years, this is not a new concept. Humans have used cold temperatures to alleviate pain, support healing, and elevate moods for centuries.

HOW DOES CRYOTHERAPY WORK?

Firstly, we need to understand what causes chronic pain. Many people struggle with chronic health issues. Often, their struggles are reminiscent of a great battle in Greek mythology between Hercules, the hero of all heroes and the strongest of men, and Hydra, a snake-like water beast with many heads.

The goddess of wisdom, Athena, gave Hercules a unique golden sword to defeat his foe, but Hydra was a deadly competitor. Every time Hercules cut off one of Hydra's heads, the seemingly immortal beast grew another two. Fortunately for Hercules, one of Hydra's heads was mortal, and when Hercules cut it off, Hydra finally died.

Hydra is an analogy for treating one symptom only to have one or more others take its place. Like the manifold heads of Hydra, various health issues affect many of us. While nipping symptoms one at a time with medicine or surgery may provide temporary relief, it does not deal with the source of the problem.

We take a pill for one health issue, another pill for a different issue, and a third to combat the side effects of the first two. But time and again, the pills only offer temporary relief. And sometimes, we have to take medication for the rest of our lives.

Our modern society mainly relies on two treatment methods in traditional medicine: biochemistry (drugs) and surgery. These treatments are lifesaving and have helped millions of people. However, in many instances, there is a price to pay, often resulting in undesirable consequences. For example, even the best surgical operations can leave scar tissue, hindering movement by making it more difficult for the different layers of muscles and connective tissue to move freely. So, much like fighting Hydra, our symptom-repression often results in more symptoms popping up.

Given our busy lives, most people are affected by some form of health problems from time to time. The symptoms can fade and recur at sporadic intervals. If they persist, we must do something to address them.

Rather than addressing the symptoms with a pill, I recommend finding a solution that treats the root cause. If we practice cold therapy effectively, there is a good chance that we can alleviate or eliminate many of the most common health problems. This belief is based not only on my personal experience and the testimonials of countless individuals but also on an ever-growing body of research in this area.

THE SCIENCE BEHIND CRYOTHERAPY

It's important to understand the science behind cryotherapy and its many benefits. One of the most notable physiological responses to cryotherapy is the release of norepinephrine into the bloodstream. This hormone neurotransmitter plays a vital role in focus, cognizance, awareness, energy, and mood. Norepinephrine also has significant positive effects on metabolism, pain, and inflammation.

A recent study showed that those who did whole-body cryotherapy for around 2 minutes at 40°F (4.4°C) three times a week for more than twelve weeks experienced a boost of norepinephrine levels in their blood by up to 300%. [1]

Restorative cold therapy can help with neurodegenerative diseases by concealing neuronal overexpression and inflammation. Cooling infants to 91.4°F (33°C) from the normal body temperature of 98.6°F (37°C) for three days after birth is used to treat hypoxic-ischemic encephalopathy, a type of brain dysfunction that arises when the brain doesn't receive enough oxygen.[2] This treatment suppresses brain damage and increases the infant's chances of survival.

A low temperature also increases adiponectin, which is a protein that helps with blood sugar administration. The cold also encourages glucose uptake similar to GLUT4 and may be used to prevent type-2 diabetes.

Sleeping in marginally colder temperatures improves baseline sleep, time spent in deep sleep, and overall sleep satisfaction. It can also enhance the production of melatonin and the administration of the circadian clock.

Cold exposure triggers the immune system in a similar way to exercise and can improve immunity. According to recent reports, healthy young people who took a daily hot-to-cold shower for thirty days did not take as much time off work due to illness—there was a 29% decrease in sick leave. However, it is important to note that being exposed to a low temperature while you are sick could make you sicker, as your immune system is already weakened.

The same applies to exercise. If you're overtraining, this could make you weaker. However, if you're working hard while remaining healthy, it will eventually strengthen your immune system. So, don't overtrain or sleep too little when you're showing evident signs of sickness.

Also, you don't need to jump straight into an ice bath to get the benefits from cold exposure. Showering under cold water for thirty seconds can help you adapt to colder temperatures. Personally, in winter, I keep the house heating off as often as possible, so I get used to lower temperatures. Small changes, like wearing one less layer in winter, are great when it comes to improving your immune system and developing resilience to physical stress.

Exposing skin to these low temperatures produces a series of physiological responses, all of which help the body repair itself. When the temperature drops, blood flow in the joints behaves similarly to blood flow in the skin. The body desires to preserve its internal core temperature by changing the peripheral or skin temperature via a vasomotor administration of the small blood vessels in the skin.

To define these medical terms, vasoconstriction is the narrowing of the blood vessels resulting from the contraction of the muscular wall of the vessels. The process is the opposite of vasodilation, which is the widening of blood vessels.

Heat loss is escalated by peripheral vasodilatation. Conversely, heat is maintained by peripheral vasoconstriction. The initial response to the application of cold is vasoconstriction involving:

- A direct and continuous constriction of the superficial blood vessels locally,
- Instant general vasoconstriction by involuntary action through the central nervous system, and
- Prolonged generalized vasoconstriction as a result of activation of the posterior hypothalamus by the cool venous blood coming back to the common circulation from the cooled skin.

If you put your finger in icy water, the tissue temperature drops instantly. When the tissue temperature reaches 59°F (15°C), reflex vasodilatation occurs, increasing the finger temperature by at least 41°F (5°C). This secondary vasodilatation has an important security function: it maintains the viability of body tissue at low temperatures.

During a cryotherapy treatment, your body also produces cold shock proteins. Cold shock proteins are liable to the metabolism of lipids or fat burning. This means your body becomes more efficient at burning fat.

Exposing your body to mild cold conditions, such as taking a cold shower or splashing cold water on your face or chest, accelerates the stimulation of the vagus nerve. The vagus nerve is the main component of the parasympathetic nervous system, which affects many crucial bodily functions, including control of mood, immune response, digestion, and heart rate. A healthy vagus nerve is essential in overall health and wellbeing.

While your body acclimates to the cold, sympathetic activity decreases, whereas parasympathetic activity increases. Mild cold exposure has been shown to drive the vagus nerve and activate cholinergic neurons through the vagus nerve course. Researchers have established that regularly exposing yourself to the cold can decrease your sympathetic 'fight or flight' response and increase parasympathetic exertion through the vagus nerve.

Inflammation is a crucial process when it comes to initiating tissue repair in the event of cell injury. However, our body goes over the top at times: the inflammatory process continues even in the absence of injury. Chronic inflammation is considered a silent killer and plays a large role in the aging process. Further, it is connected with multiple chronic and complex health conditions such as Alzheimer's disease, atherosclerosis, cardiovascular disease, type II diabetes, and cancer.

To highlight the harmful impact of inflammation, a detailed study concluded that "high levels of pro-inflammatory markers in the blood and other tissues are often detected in older individuals and predict the risk of cardiovascular diseases, frailty, multimorbidity, and decline of physical and cognitive function."[3]

The study detected only one biomarker that forecasts survival and level of cognition: low inflammation. And guess what reduces inflammation?— Norepinephrine.

WHAT ARE THE POTENTIAL SIDE EFFECTS OF CRYOTHERAPY?

While cryotherapy can alleviate unwanted pain and nerve irritation, it can sometimes create abnormal sensations, such as numbness or tingling. Further, it can sometimes bring short-term redness and irritation to the skin. Some of the side effects noted in local cryotherapy patients include respiratory problems, frostbite, and joint or muscle pain.[4],[5]

Potential side effects noted in those who undertake whole-body cryotherapy can include the following: headaches, hypertension, dizziness, joint or muscle pain, anxiety, respiratory problems, long-lasting coldness, urticaria, an increased heartbeat, palpitations, insomnia, bowel sounds, bloating, muscle contraction, and shivering[6].

Cold water submersion before exercise decreases maximum power output, heart rate, and overall performance. There is no logical reason for a cold water plunge immediately before exercise; on the contrary, you should ensure that your muscles are warmed up to prevent injuries. Some studies show that cold therapy alleviates muscle soreness after exercise, but others find no significant benefit. Personally, I believe that cold therapy works extremely well for increased recovery. Why else would the New York Knicks basketball team and sportsmen like LeBron James, Kobe Bryant, Floyd Mayweather, and Cristiano Ronaldo swear by cryotherapy to manage sports injury and muscle recovery?

The potential side-effects outlined below are short-lived and tend to occur when you do not practice cryotherapy frequently.

Post-workout cold water therapy can attenuate the anabolic signaling and long-term acclimations in muscle to strength training. It is similar to antioxidants that block the ROS (Reactive Oxygen Species) and inflammation, which you need in some volume to make the body adapt.

Cold exposure burns calories and accelerates your metabolic rate, but it can also make you hungrier. It doesn't matter how much fat you're burning if you make up for this by over-eating. Furthermore, although the cold doesn't tend to directly decrease immunity, if you over-expose yourself to it or become stressed out, you will risk lowering your thyroid functioning and, in turn, slow down your metabolism.

If a localized cold pack or ice is left on the skin for too long, it can cause skin damage (including frostbite). Therefore, localized cold therapy should never be employed for longer than thirty minutes, and the skin should be examined during treatment.

Generally, a quick cold shower, or even an ice bath for two to three minutes, isn't enough to cause negative side effects. Usually, the side effects occur as a result of chronic overexposure, other stressors, or getting exposed to the cold when your immune system is weak.

Whole-body cryotherapy should not be practiced for longer than five minutes (typical treatment sessions last two to three minutes). Whole-body cryotherapy causes suppressed heart rate, accelerated blood pressure, and lowered respiration. The patient's vital signs and moods should be monitored before, during, and after treatment. Oxygen levels inside the chamber should also be monitored.

The patient should ensure that their clothing and skin are completely dry before entering a cryotherapy chamber. Also, metal or jewelry should be removed. Lastly, sensitive body parts should be covered using a face cover, ear coverings, gloves, and socks or slippers. Frostbite can occur when a patient does not proceed with the proper caution when entering a cryotherapy chamber.

After reading the science behind cryotherapy and its possible side effects, you can probably tell that this book intends to show how a normal person can adapt and enhance their body using cold exposure with little effort.

Many hormetic stressors, like fasting and exposure to heat and cold, are ideal when it comes to disease prevention, not treatment. Keep up these practices while you are healthy, and they will protect you from illness.

The simplest and best way to start is to take a cold shower for just twenty to thirty seconds. Your immediate response might be to tense up, but this can be even more stressful. Also, it will create a spontaneous habit – one of always tensing and never getting used to the cold. Instead, submit to the cold and don't overreact. Just stand there and think about what is happening to your body. The key is not to focus on feeling the cold or on your pain. Rather, imagine a more pleasant sensation is making contact with your body.

Taking ice baths or swimming outdoors in winter is a stronger form of cold thermogenesis. It's healthy to do this at least once or twice a month.

Combining ice baths or cold exposure with hot saunas is a fantastic way to boost the effectiveness of both. This will be explored in detail in Chapter 7.

Exposure to acute cold and rewarming triggers autophagy. Autophagy, defined by Priya Khorana from Columbia University, is the body's way of cleaning out damaged cells to regenerate newer, healthier cells.

"Auto" means self, and "phagy" means eat. Therefore, the literal meaning of autophagy is "self-eating."

Cold exposure also encourages lymph flow and circulation. If you have cardiovascular problems or disease, avoid subjecting your body to rapid alterations in temperature, as this can be harmful.

If you're still not fully convinced by cold exposure yet, look at the testimonials of those who practice it. Cryotherapy has been around for centuries.

Hippocrates, the father of medicine, is believed to have documented the benefits of cold exposure when used to treat bleeding, swelling, and pain way back in 400B.C. Since then, physicians and scientists have strongly supported the use of cold therapy in suppressing chronic pain.

In a 1697 brief to Prince William, Duke of Devonshire, Doctor John Floyer gave his approval regarding the use of cold baths to cure and alleviate chronic pain linked to rickets and rheumatisms[6].

In 1978, Dr. Yamauchi coined the phrase "whole body cryotherapy." He used the modality to help his patients manage the pain of rheumatoid arthritis by freezing their skin. After experiencing positive results, he and his partner developed cryotherapy chambers.

Today, general physicians and physical therapists prescribe cryotherapy to alleviate chronic aches and pains, especially due to its simplicity and low cost.

After reading the scientific testimonials, I trust you now believe in the magic of cryotherapy. Yet, to this day, the idea that cold therapy plays a vital role in overcoming health problems is still overlooked. Indeed, Wim Hof's achievements were long considered to be scientifically impossible. It was only after the first Radboud University study in 2011 that beliefs and attitudes towards cold therapy started to change. This study addressed the fact that Hof could freely influence his autonomic nervous system – something which had previously been considered impossible. This groundbreaking method, published in PNAS and Nature, revised biology textbooks and evoked the curiosity of scientists.

So, to bring revolution to our bodies and our society, we must educate ourselves about cold exposure.

In upcoming chapters, we will focus on three methods of cryotherapy:

1. Cold water therapy.
2. Cryotherapy machines.
3. Outdoor cold therapy.

I will also explain how anyone on any budget can benefit from cryotherapy. Furthermore, I will help you focus on developing good daily habits as I encourage you to take one step at a time, as cold therapy is all about easing in gently.

GETTING TO GRIPS WITH SOME CRYO-TERMINOLOGY

Before we further explore the benefits of cold exposure, let's take a look at some of the terminology:

Hormesis

The sensory system is complex. Receptors in the skin respond immediately when the body is exposed to the cold. If the response to this is insufficient to maintain the body's core temperature, receptors in the brain note a fall in temperature, inducing a harsher reaction to the cold.

The term hormesis represents the paradoxical adaptation that makes animals stronger if they are exposed to environmental stressors for short periods of time. If they were exposed to these stressors for a long time, however, they would prove lethal. Everything, including cold water, can be harmful at high enough doses. However, as hormesis proves, it can have beneficial results.

Throughout this book, I present discussions of the results cold-water therapies can have on the central nervous system. The benefits may result from the subsequent changes that occur within the central nervous system.

System Wind-up

The term 'System Wind-Up' was introduced in a report by Michael Ridgway. Ridgway claims that system wind-up happens when there are "[...] boundless unhappy signals (negative signals/toxic inputs) resulting from unhelpful thoughts, behaviors, and feelings." These unhappy inputs are sent to the subconscious brain and spinal cord, which has a negative impact on the overall structure of the body. System wind-up is also regularly referred to as central sensitization.

I mention this point to help you understand why pain and suffering happen in the human body.

The Mammalian Diving Reflex

The Mammalian Diving Reflex is another inborn biological response to cold immersion. As the name implies, all mammals show this response, even humans, albeit to a weaker degree. This reflex exists to increase the time that animals can endure being submerged underwater by lowering the need for respiration.

2

THE PHYSICAL AND MENTAL BENEFITS OF COLD EXPOSURE

The ability of homo sapiens to adapt to the cold and heat has been key to our survival. It is believed that humans evolved from a tropical environment. For the most part, our bodies are not well suited to the cold. After all, we are not covered in fur, nor do we have thick hair all over our bodies. The fact that we can dwell in cold climates is a result of man-made habitat adaptations like clothing and shelter.

Humans naturally keep their core temperature remarkably constant so that the temperature of the heart, brain, and other central organs seldom rises or falls more than a few degrees above or below 98,6°F (37°C). One of the ways we achieve a constant core temperature is through conscious protective measures such as putting on protective clothing or entering sheltered accommodation when our sensory system detects exposure to cold temperatures.

As I mentioned in the previous chapter, cold water has been considered a superhero and a supervillain for centuries. It is believed to have both beneficial and harmful effects. However, the use of the cold as a therapeutic agent has a long history. The Edwin Smith Papyrus, the earliest known medical text, dated 3,500 B.C., supports the use of the cold as a therapy.

Ancient China, Greece, Egypt, and Rome documented the medicinal uses of hydrotherapy. Various reports from the time refer to hydrotherapy as 'the water remedy' or 'hydropathy.'

In 1961, Irving S. Cooper (1922-1985), a talented neurosurgeon, created the first closed cryoprobe system and guided the modern era of cryogenic surgery.

WHO WILL BENEFIT FROM COLD EXPOSURE?

1. People who want to lose weight.

Humans typically possess a small amount of active brown fat tissue, also known as brown adipose tissue. Unlike white fat, which stores energy, brown fat helps to burn calories and utilize energy. Its prime function is to warm up the body. Adipose tissue is considered 'good' fat because it speeds up your metabolism.

White adipocytes, or white fat cells, have a single lipid droplet, but brown adipocytes consist of many tiny lipid droplets and many iron-carrying mitochondria. It is this high iron volume that gives brown fat its dark red color.

Brown fat contains more capillaries than white fat. This is because of its higher oxygen consumption. Brown fat also has several unmyelinated nerves, providing sympathetic stimulation to the fat cells.

Studies[1] reveal that cold exposure increases brown adipose tissue activity that leads to increased calorie spending. Researchers concluded that repeated cold exposures might be a suitable and cost-effective approach to addressing the obesity epidemic. According to preliminary research, a lack of brown adipose tissue has been linked with obesity.

Cold exposure increases quivering and non-quivering thermogenesis. These processes accelerate calorie expenditure. Exposure to cold temperatures leads to improved levels of adiponectin – a protein that accelerates fat burning. Low levels of adiponectin relate to obesity.

Overweight people who are regularly exposed to the cold can train their bodies to turn white fat into energy via brown fat.

A 2011 study by Marken-Lichtenbelt[2] shows that brown adipose tissue can be activated by the cold. Brown fat became activated when temperatures dropped to 64.4°F (18°C). This activation is designed to bring the body temperature back up to normal. As the temperature drops, more brown adipose tissue is activated.

2. People who suffer from frequent inflammation.

Inflammation is a part of our body's protection mechanism and plays a vital role in healing. When the body senses an intruder, it initiates a biological response in order to remove it. The intruder could be an external body, such as an irritant, a spike, or a pathogen. Pathogens include viruses, bacteria, and other organisms, all of which bring about infections.

Sometimes, the body incorrectly perceives its own cells or tissues as harmful. This response can lead to autoimmune diseases. Experts believe that inflammation may cause a wide range of chronic diseases. For example, metabolic syndrome, which consists of type 2 diabetes, obesity, and heart disease. People with these symptoms often have higher levels of inflammatory markers in their bodies.

Cold immersions have been scientifically proven to counteract the side effects of muscle overuse, such as pain, soreness, and tightness. When we submerge in cold water, we compress a lot of the blood vessels, which helps to increase adiponectin – a protein that fights inflammation.

In addition, direct cold exposure can numb nerve endings and, in turn, act as a pain reliever. Many professional athletes use an ice bath after their workouts and competitions for this very reason.

Another study established that exercising in a cold environment reduced the inflammatory response observed in regular temperature environments[3]. However, this same study found that exercising in the cold for an extended time can increase the inflammatory response, so discretion is advised.

The disadvantages of using cryotherapy to treat inflammation:

- Ice burn
- Inhibits muscle function

- Cryotherapy-induced nerve injuries

3. People who want longevity.

Some consider cold water exposure to be the fountain of everlasting youth! Showering in very hot water can strip away some of the crucial oils that help your skin look youthful. Although it feels nice, hot water is not always a friend to your skin.

The downside of hot showers for your skin:

- Hot water can dry out and irritate your skin if it damages the keratin cells in your epidermis, preventing them from locking in moisture.
- Hot water aggravates skin conditions like eczema.
- Hot water can cause the skin to itch when mast cells release histamine onto the skin.

Your skin is the largest organ in your body. Heat damages this crucial barrier and can make you look older. In contrast, cold water tightens the epidermis, closing pores, reducing puffiness, and helping your skin look brighter and more youthful for longer.

Improved longevity through cold exposure could be due to hormesis, as discussed earlier. Alternatively, increased longevity from cold exposure may be due to the regulation of genes, such as DAF-16 and TRPA-1. Up until now, however, no studies have been done on humans.

We know that cold water reduces stress, puts you in a better mood, helps your body burn fat, keeps you looking youthful, boosts your immune system, and helps you deal with the trials of everyday life. All of this, in turn, keeps you healthier for longer. Some studies[4] even propose that cold water can improve the survival rates of various types of cancer. However, none of these tests were done on humans.

4. People who have a weak immune system.

The worldwide Covid-19 pandemic has shown how important preventative care is. What you consume and how much you exercise is also important. However, nutrients aren't the only means to boost your immunity.

Continual cold exposure makes cortisol levels fall. As a result of a rise in endorphins, your body can commit more energy to revitalize your immune system and, in turn, combat invaders.

5. People who have insomnia or poor sleep quality.

For those suffering from irregular sleep patterns or insomnia, adopting a cold exposure habit before bed and introducing cryotherapy as part of your healthy lifestyle routine may help enhance sleep.

As previously mentioned, cryotherapy or cold exposure exposes your body to cold temperatures for short periods of time to enhance the production of norepinephrine. This hormone influences your sleep/wake cycles and activates your rapid eye movement (REM) sleep. The release of endorphins may result in an energy upliftment which is followed by a state of tranquility. Filtered, oxygen-rich blood moves back through your body, which may help to reduce inflammation and pain. These reactions can work together to help you fall asleep and experience deeper levels of REM sleep, as they help you remain asleep for longer.

6. People who suffer from chronic pain.

Cold therapy is frequently used to help relieve pain from muscle or joint injury. Cold treatment lessens blood flow to the damaged area. This slows the rate of inflammation and decreases the risk of swelling and tissue damage.

Cold therapy also immobilizes sore tissues, acting as a local anesthetic, and slows down the pain messages being transferred to the brain. Ice can help treat an inflamed and swollen joint or muscle. It is most successful when applied within 48 hours of an injury.

Sports injuries are frequently caused by a direct impact, overuse, or the application of force that is greater than the body part can structurally resist. Common injuries include sprains, strains, bruises, and joint injuries.

R.I.C.E. stands for Rest, Ice, Compression, and Elevation. Following these simple steps after sustaining an injury can help you recover more quickly and get back to day-to-day activities.

Rest

Rest the injured or affected area. Avoid moving it and try to keep weight off it. Use braces, canes, splints, or crutches when available. Avoid weight-bearing activities for between 24 to 48 hours. Continued use of a moderate or severely sprained joint can delay healing, increase pain, or even worsen the injury. With a mild sprain, activity can generally be resumed after 24 to 48 hours of rest.

Ice

To help reduce pain and swelling during the first 48 hours of injury, ice the affected area for twenty minutes at a time every three to four hours. Use an ice pack wrapped in a towel. If you don't have an ice pack handy, use a bag of frozen corn, peas, or other vegetables. Try not to ice the injured area for more than 20 minutes at a time, as this may cause additional tissue damage.

Side effects of localized ice treatment:

You may experience numbness, tingling, redness, and skin irritation. However, these side effects are most often temporary. See your doctor if these symptoms persist for longer than 24 hours.

Compression

Compress the injured area. Using a flexible medical bandage, wrap the area to help reduce swelling and internal bleeding. The wrap should be comfortable, so make sure you have good circulation. Some signs that the bandage is too tight include tingling, numbness, coolness, increased pain, and/or swelling. If you think you need to use the wrap for more than 48 to 72 hours, consult a medical expert, as you may have more serious issues that require prompt medical attention.

Elevation

Elevate the injured area. Raise the injured body part above your heart level. This will allow gravity to transfer fluids away from the injured area. Experts say it is beneficial to elevate the area for between two to three hours a day.

7. People who suffer from Arthritis.

Arthritis is a disorder that is identified by pain in the joints caused by inflammation. The pain can have several causes, as there are two types of arthritis: osteoarthritis and rheumatoid arthritis. Osteoarthritis is caused when the cartilage that cushions the ends of the bones in your joints deteriorates. Rheumatoid arthritis is caused when your immune system mistakenly sends antibodies to the lining of your joints, attacking the tissue surrounding the joint. Arthritis is a very common disorder affecting millions of people globally.

To reduce the symptoms of arthritis, many physicians prescribe medication such as painkillers and non-steroidal anti-inflammatory drugs (NSAIDs). However, seeking relief with the help of drugs is not without risk —medicines can have severe side effects. Fortunately, options are available for those who wish to manage arthritis naturally, as cold exposure can relieve the symptoms related to arthritis.

The cold can help reduce pain, swelling, and muscle spasms. Arthritic joints feel healthier and can function better when there is less pain and swelling. Also, the cold reduces swelling through *vasoconstriction*, which is the constriction of the blood vessels. When blood vessels shrink, blood flow is reduced, and the release of *histamine* is blocked. Blocking histamine reduces the feeling of pain.

Cold also triggers sensory receptors that help to block the transmission of pain stimulation that travel along the nerves. This temporarily enhances a person's pain threshold in the affected area.

8. People who suffer from dementia.

Researchers from Cambridge University have revealed that cold water swimming may safeguard the brain from degenerative diseases like dementia. Professor Giovanna Mallucci, who runs the UK Dementia Research Institute's Centre at the University of Cambridge, says this discovery could point researchers toward new medical treatments that may help to keep dementia at bay[5].

A medically induced hypothermic state has a long history in clinical settings and is frequently used to help people recover from cardiac activities and head injuries. After all, it has long been accepted that being kept in a cooler environment gives someone recovering from surgery or a traumatic injury a better chance of survival, as most bacteria and viruses do not thrive in colder conditions.

In terms of brain health, when the body is cool, it can protect the brain against the loss of cells and aid healthy synapses—the connection points between brain cells that transfer electrical and chemical impulses. Healthy synapses are important to keep your brain functioning as it should.

Although there is no conclusive evidence as to whether or not frequently inducing a decreased body temperature through cold exposure can prevent neurodegenerative decline, there appears to be a connection between swimming in cold water and higher levels of protective RBM3, a cold-induced RNA binding protein[6].

9. People who have Alzheimer's disease.

Finding treatments for Alzheimer's has proven to be extremely difficult. The disease is characterized by the development of two distinct pathologies in the brain:

- Senile plaques, made up of β-amyloid situated predominantly between neuronal cells that gather in normal aging without dementia.
- Tangles appear from tau aggregation, forming tiny toxic, pathological oligomers and then filaments within neuronal cells. These aggregates are connected to both clinical dementia and radiology abnormalities generally used for diagnosis.

We still know very little about what activates the accumulation of these proteins. However, we do know that the disease can develop decades before any clinical symptoms appear. There is also little understanding about how the unusual processing of the proteins which give rise to β-amyloid plaques and tangles are connected and which comes first. There are strong connections between clinical decline and the largely homogenous growth of the tangle pathology throughout the brain.

It has been known for some time that the connection between clinical decline and β-amyloid pathology is feebler than for the tau aggregation pathology. In recent years, this has been affirmed using particular ligands that allow the two forms of pathology to be envisioned in living patients using PET imaging.

Thermogenesis is the process where our body produces heat to keep warm. So, if we dissect cold thermogenesis, this will completely start the process. Upon exposure to colder temperatures, your body must work diligently to control your core body temperature and nurture homeostasis. Keeping our body warm to generate this heat burns more calories.

Therefore, the evidence is fascinating and calls for further investigation of the potential benefits of heat adaption and passive heat therapy for patients with neurodegenerative diseases.

10. Cold exposure for children.

It is strictly prohibited for children to practice extreme cold exposure. If parents wish their children to benefit from cold exposure, they can tell them about the treatment and gently introduce them to the cold exposure process with mild cold showers.

However, cryotherapy can be used to treat certain conditions and injuries in children, including the treatment of viral warts, sprains, and inflammation.

Treating warts with cryotherapy involves freezing them using a very cold substance like liquid nitrogen. The liquid nitrogen treatment normally takes less than a minute. This type of cryotherapy can be done in a doctor's office.

When cold therapy is most effective

Patients who are unsure whether they should practice cold therapy should consult their doctor or physiotherapist for advice. Cold therapy can provide benefits in the following scenarios:

- For 24-78 hours following injury or orthopedic surgery
- To decrease muscle spasms
- To decrease swelling in arthritic joints
- To decrease pain in arthritic joints

CRYOTHERAPY CAN BE USED TO TREAT SOME TYPES OF CANCER

The national cancer institute released a paper[7] that reports that cryotherapy, in the form of cryosurgery, can treat certain types of cancer. These include:

- skin cancers, including basal cell and squamous cell carcinomas
- skin lesions from AIDS-related Kaposi sarcoma
- retinoblastoma
- liver cancer that is confined to the liver

- non-small cell lung cancer
- early-stage prostate cancer
- bone cancer, mostly chondrosarcoma

Cryosurgery can also be used to treat these non-cancerous conditions:

- Abnormal cell changes in the cervix that can turn into cervical cancer, known as cervical intraepithelial neoplasia or cervical precancer.
- Benign bone tumors, such as enchondroma, giant cell tumor, aneurysmal bone cyst, and chondroblastoma.
- Skin growths called actinic keratoses that can turn into cancer.

Cryosurgery freezes tissue, causing cells in the treated area to die.

THE DANGERS OF COLD EXPOSURE

Essentially, practicing cryotherapy is safe if you're healthy, and, upon consultation with your doctor, it can be safely practiced even if you have some health concerns. After all, cold exposure can assist in healing and relieving ailments and symptoms, as I detailed throughout this chapter. If you're not used to the cold, prolonged and repetitive cold exposure can cause negative side effects. That's why it's important to build your endurance slowly.

Hormetic stressors like heat, cold, and fasting are most effective as disease *prevention*, not treatment. It would be best if you started doing them while you're healthy, as a shield against illness and poor health in the future.

The easiest and best way to start practicing cold exposure is to take a cold shower. Just 30 to 60 seconds of cold water is not too difficult a ritual to get into, but you will reap the benefits. Your first reaction might be to tense up but resist this urge and try to stay relaxed. Pay attention to how your body responds. The key is not to focus on feeling the cold or discomfort.

PRECAUTIONS WHEN ENTERING COLD BODIES OF WATER

Although the cold usually causes our heart rate and breathing to drop, the shock of cold immersion can cause an initial, substantial rise in heart rate and blood pressure, which can cause heart attacks and strokes in those with underlying conditions. Cold immersion can also cause rapid breathing and a gasp reflex that can lead to drowning if water is inhaled.

Only take a dip with others who are experienced with cold water therapy and check for potential hazards in advance. Search for individuals or active cold therapy group near you. Before diving into cold water, speak to your general physician.

3

A COLD SHOWER A DAY KEEPS THE DOCTOR AWAY

"You gain strength, courage, and confidence by every experience in which you really stop to look fear in the face. You are able to say to yourself, 'I have lived through this horror. I can take the next thing that comes along.' You must do the thing you think you cannot do." — *Eleanor Roosevelt*

ARE YOU AFRAID OF GETTING COLD?

Now that we know that taking a cold shower is good for your body and mind, why are we still so afraid of cold showers? Maybe it's because we've been conditioned to desire comfort and warmth, and that warmth has become a necessity.

I've always been curious about the difference between bathing in cold water versus hot water. Before I discovered the benefits of cryotherapy, the thought of having a cold shower every single day was hardly an exciting prospect as I loved hot water. In fact, I was always a little concerned that using cold water might lead to various problems—will I feel as clean? Will I develop a cough or a cold? I was never entirely sure if washing my hair with cold water would be as beneficial as washing it with lukewarm or hot water.

I used to be one of those people who preferred standing under a rushing hot shower, and I would stay there until my skin became lobster-red. There was something compulsive about the feeling of searing warmth all over. When I first heard people talking about the advantages of cold showers, I was doubtful – I could hardly muster the courage to wade into the sea on a hot day.

Although I used to be slightly wary of cold exposure, I have always been health conscious. Conscious living and questioning the status quo is a way of life for me.

Also, when I decide to try something new, it must have some clear and obvious benefits. So, when I first heard about cryotherapy, I was pleased to see it had many supporters, all of whom testified to its physical and mental health benefits.

I wanted to put the claims to the test, so I began my initial '7 Day Cold Shower Challenge.'

When my wife and I moved into our first house, the shower system was old and needed replacing. When looking for a new shower, there were several options to choose from. I made a conscious decision to choose a shower system that allowed me to isolate the cold water. Some modern shower systems do not allow you to run cold water only. If you have one of those systems but are serious about starting cold showers, then you may want to consider changing your shower. It will come at a cost in the short term but think about the long-term benefits.

Another factor that inspired me to try cold showers was the fact that I love to set challenges for myself. I used to create short daily workout challenges. I realized that this would be the perfect time to combine my workouts with a new challenge. Author of the best-selling book, Atomic Habits, James Clear has defined combining two or more positive habits together as "habit stacking":

"One of the best ways to develop a new habit is to recognize a present habit you already do every day and then stack your new habit on top."

I decided to stack the habit of daily exercise with my new habit of cold showers. Initially, my goal was to take cold showers for seven days. I will go into more detail about habit stacking in Chapter 6.

SLOW AND STEADY WINS THE RACE

One principle I always keep in mind whenever I start doing anything new is to *ease in gently*. Instead of jumping into the cold water directly, I first started with my normal shower and gradually turned the hot water down until the shower was warm. I then turned the hot water down a little more until the water was cool. Finally, I turned the hot water off completely. I was unable to stay in for very long. Nothing prepared me for the biting cold! I gasped, tensed up, waited a few seconds, and then jumped out! I stepped out from under the cold water after 10 seconds—it was instinctive. My body wants to be comfortable.

Only later did I realize that it's not good to tense up and overreact. It was much more beneficial when I learned to submit to the cold. Take the time to be in the moment and *experience* what is happening to your body. Don't focus on the cold or discomfort.

Never stay under cold water for so long that you cannot stop shivering. If you find yourself in this situation, you've been exposed to the cold for too long, which is unhealthy, doing your body more harm than good. While some can withstand cold showers for five to ten minutes, it's fine if you can only manage as little as ten to thirty seconds. Start where you can and gradually increase your exposure time. Above all else, listen to your body.

I'd love to say having a cold shower became easier the next day, but it was still a struggle. It was a mental battle for the next few days. By day four, it started becoming a little easier as my body was starting to get conditioned for the daily habit. In the first few days, the mistake I made was holding my breath and gasping, and not staying relaxed. I learned to prepare myself by taking a few deep breaths before going in and breathing through the initial shock of the cold. Taking those deep breaths before entering the cold shower definitely helped.

Breathing can have a huge impact on how our bodies adjust to the cold. The body's initial reaction to the shock is to hyperventilate; our breathing becomes quick and irregular. Deep breathing through the initial shock will send signals to the brain, which calms us down. Deep breathing and repeated exposure to the cold can suppress the shiver response and prevent the gasping that you may be tempted to succumb to during your first few cold showers.

Here are some benefits I gained from my first week of cold showers:

I was less stressed.

When you get under that cold water, it's almost impossible to think of anything else. At that moment, nothing else matters. Stress melts away. Those 30 seconds seemed to last forever. If hot showers send you to a place of profound thought, a cold shower makes you think of nothing—other than the fact that you are in a cold shower! Once you come to terms with this, something interesting starts to happen.

As I practiced my breathing techniques, I started to relax. I eased my tense shoulders. My breathing slowed, and I became composed.

I became more productive.

After every cold shower, I felt fresh and revitalized. I felt like I had started the day off on the right foot and found myself being extremely productive. Before taking cold showers, I was never an early bird, and I always felt lethargic in the mornings.

I had more energy and felt like I could achieve anything. I was setting ambitious goals and working through my To-Do list like never before. This feeling alone cemented my belief in the power of cold showers.

There were other benefits, too. A cold shower worked wonders for my sore muscles. Also, my hair became extra smooth and shiny.

The week had been a success, so I convinced myself that I would continue to take cold showers every morning.

I was becoming addicted to it because of the way it made me feel.

After one month, I started to see the following physical and mental changes:

1. Mentally, cold showers improved my willpower and self-belief, filling me with the confidence and motivation to set bigger goals for my life and, in turn, adopt even more positive habits.
2. My body became accustomed to cold temperatures. In the middle of winter, where

the temperatures could drop to around 20ºF (-06C), I walk outdoors in shorts and a t-shirt. I get some strange looks and people asking, "Aren't you cold?"

3. Please be aware that there are risks to being outdoors in sub-zero temperatures without the right clothing and shoes. Unless you are in peak health and have allowed yourself to become accustomed to the cold over time, don't attempt this. You could get sick with a cough, cold, or flu because the cold can further diminish a weakened immune response. You could also suffer from hyperthermia.

4. My muscle and joint pain started to improved. My muscles and joints became less stiff and achy. Further, I noticed that my recovery time after working out was becoming shorter. I started exercising five times a week, with very little soreness after sessions.

5. My immune system was improving. To my delight, I have not become ill since I started taking cold showers.

6. My energy levels were higher and remained consistent throughout the day. I no longer had the morning lethargy and the mid-afternoon slump that I used to experience.

7. It allowed me to reconnect with nature. I feel short spells of absolute bliss, joy, gratitude, and love during a cold shower. This is me reconnecting with nature and my inner being. I feel like I'm tapping into my inner fire and uncovering my true nature.

For many, the idea of taking a cold shower seems ridiculous. Despite this, an enthusiastic movement exists where people are praising the benefits of cold showers.

As I have mentioned, sports professionals and athletes have frequently used cold water to cure sore muscles.

Other physical benefits of cold exposure include increased weight loss and healthier skin tone. There is also evidence that cold showers can help with your mental health. One research report published in *Medical Hypotheses* shows that cold showers could be used to relieve the symptoms of depression[1].

If you're keen to give cold therapy a try without the expense that comes with using cryotherapy machines, cold showers are a great way to ease yourself in.

You do not have to be a superhero or extraordinarily brave to take a cold shower. If I can do it, anybody can.

HOW DO YOU GET STARTED WITH COLD EXPOSURE?

You need to prepare your mind before you take the plunge.

The aim is ultimately to make yourself love a cold bath or shower, despite initially regarding it as something you do unwillingly for the sake of your well-being. Changing your mindset is immensely important, and it takes some time to master.

Chapter 5 goes into greater detail to explain how we can master any circumstance if we have the right mindset. It also explores how not all stress is equal. In fact, there is such a thing as *good* stress—and cold exposure is one of the triggers of good stress.

Cold Exposure: Beginner

Here are some easy behaviors that a complete beginner can use to get started with cold therapy.

1. Wash your face with cold water.

Stepping straight into a cold shower can be daunting if you've never done it before. To ease yourself into it and to get your body conditioned for the initial shock that comes with cold exposure, start by splashing your face with cold water in the morning for a few days. You could also splash your chest with a little cold water.

2. Gradually go from a warm to a cold shower.

An easy way to get started is to begin with a regular warm shower and then gradually decrease the temperature until you reach the point where you are only running cold water. This method takes away the initial shock of the cold by easing you in gently. After a few days, you can reduce your time under the hot water and speed up the transition to cold water only.

Stretch the cold phase of the shower to last for twenty to thirty seconds (this will feel like a lifetime at first). Over the next few weeks, work your way up gradually to two to three minutes of cold water. After a month, you may even skip the 'warm' part of the shower altogether.

Here is an example of a warm-to-cold water timetable that you can use to ease into the cold shower routine.

Week 1 – 30 seconds of cold water
Week 2 – 1 minute of cold water
Week 3 – 1 ½ minutes of cold water

Week 4 – 2 minutes of cold water
Week 5 and beyond – increase your time until you're showering in cold water only.

3. The wet towel method.

If any of the above methods don't appeal to you, or you want a less startling way to kick-start your cold exposure, try this method.

After you take a warm bath or shower, have a cold, wet towel on hand (not soaking wet, just damp) and wrap it around large areas of your body. For example, your legs, back, and chest.

Doing this gives a gentle introduction to the actual cold shower. It's not an overly enjoyable experience either. You don't have to overdo it, though – just try it a few times until the sensation becomes familiar.

4. The 'three-second' rule.

Start counting down from three seconds and then turn the cold water tap on. Do not hesitate – just do it. The more you think about it, the more your mind will try and justify why you should *not* be doing it.

Imagine a roller coaster. The scariest roller coasters are those that go up to the top really slowly. By the time you are at the summit, you are likely freaking out! There would be far less apprehension if you were on a roller coaster that just zipped you to the top and over the summit without the slow build-up. You'd hardly have time to think about it.

The same goes with cold showers. The more time you spend thinking about taking one, the more anxious you become and the less likely you are to try it. Thankfully, the 3-second rule will help you through this.

5. <u>Getting stronger.</u>

Continue lengthening the time you spend under the cold water until you become an expert at the 10-minute mark. Once you get to this level, you will feel amazing!

Have you ever seen a weightlifter before he does a heavy lift? He will focus his mind on the task at hand. Like the weightlifter, you should be as focused and calm as possible. When you step into the cold shower, remain calm. To steadily improve your performance, attempt the highest degree of cold exposure that you can manage, all while remaining as calm as possible.

Once you get out of the water, notice the sensations you experience. Your body may continue to shiver as it recovers but be sure to stay calm and trust yourself.

Staying calm while you slowly warm up is as crucial as being calm while experiencing the cold.

How cold should a cold shower be?

The average temperature for cold tap water differs depending on the season and where you live. In the northern hemisphere, water in buried water pipes will be between 45 - 55 °F (7°C - 13°C). At this temperature, cold tap water should be cold enough to kick-start your cold shower routine. If you live in a warm climate, you may need to use a cold plunge pool or bathtub with ice to cool the water.

Cold Exposure: Intermediate

If you feel comfortable with cold showers and are determined to keep going, you're ready for the next level.

Fill a bathtub or plunge pool with cold water. Start by submerging yourself for two minutes, then gradually increase this time over the next few times. If you feel uncomfortable, keep your hands out of the water but try to advance to the point where you are fully submerged up to your neck.

Cold Exposure: Extreme level, full-body immersion

Fill a bucket or small tub with ice and water. Try to place each hand and arm in the ice for between thirty seconds and one minute, but this is not mandatory. The submersion time can vary between several seconds to two minutes initially. Do the same with your feet and lower legs.

Next, fill your bathtub or plunge pool with ice and water. Climb into the tub and try and stay in for a few seconds at least. Every time you do it, increase your time. Always listen to your body.

You could also fill a chest freezer to three-quarters with cold water and ice.

IMPORTANT: ALWAYS ENSURE THAT THE FREEZER IS UNPLUGGED BEFORE YOU GET IN.

You may need to seal the internal joints of the freezer to ensure that there are no leaks.

Full-body immersion leaves me feeling great

Trust me, after doing the full-body plunge you will feel supercharged.

A 2016 study[2] found that athletes who used ice baths to recover after athletic events experienced optimal results after soaking in water between 50 to 59 °F (10 and 15 °C) for 10 to 15 minutes.

What are the risks of full-body immersion?

- People with cardiovascular disease or high blood pressure should check with their doctors before attempting extreme cold exposure.
- Hypothermia is a very real risk for anyone who stays in cold water too long.
- Don't attempt any outdoor cold exposure practices on your own.

As with any lifestyle change, when you start something new, it can take time to see results.

When I first started taking ice baths, I thought they were tough. However, I pushed through and broke my own self-limiting beliefs. Now, I take a cold shower most days, and I practice full-body immersion at least once a week.

Every day, you have two choices: stop taking cold showers and go back to the way things were or keep taking them and continue to benefit physically and mentally. Every time you feel like quitting, keep telling yourself, *"Just one more day... one more time!"* Cryotherapy, a cold shower, or full immersion in ice water is more of a mental battle than a physical one. Remember, your body will always want to give up before your mind does. Keep going.

"The secret to getting ahead is getting started." — Mark Twain

4

TAKE IT TO THE NEXT LEVEL

"Learn something new. Try something different. Convince yourself that you have no limits." — *Brian Tracy*

If you feel comfortable with cold showers and decide to take your cold therapy journey to another level, you can try cryotherapy chambers. For those who have been practicing cold exposure 'at home,' cryotherapy chambers offer a really different cold therapy experience.

You may also feel ready to try immersing yourself in natural bodies of water like lakes, rivers, or the sea. We will investigate all of these cold exposure methods in more detail in this chapter.

CRYO MACHINES

During my first cryotherapy session, I was asked to take my clothes off down to my underwear. I was given gloves, socks, and shoes to wear. The cryo-chamber, which looked like a straight-standing tanning booth, was in the middle of the room.

I would be lying if I said I was not startled by the immediate cold. My head was positioned outside the chamber, so I could still see everything around me. Also, the chamber was not locked so that I could exit at any time. I was told that almost every first-timer struggles to last a minute. I did not tell them about my previous cold exposure experience. Perhaps that is what helped me complete my first session successfully.

Was the chamber as cold as the temperatures I experienced during my outdoor cold-water dips? No. *It was even colder!* The instructor told me that the temperature for beginners is usually around -185 °F (-85 °C) and it can go down to -212 °F (-100 °C), depending on how one's body responds to the treatment.

I felt supercharged when I stepped out of the chamber. It really was a great experience.

What are cryo machines, and how do they work?

The phrase "Cryotherapy Machine" refers to a wide range of products that consists of cryotherapy chambers, cryo saunas, and localized cryotherapy units.

One can categorize cryogenic machines based on their technology, cooling procedure, characteristics, and pricing.

A cryo sauna covers the whole body, except the head, and typically works on liquid nitrogen technology. It is a popular alternative to ice baths. The machine steadily lowers the body's temperature over a period of one to three minutes.

Cryo saunas were designed to create a more relaxing cold therapy experience. After all, unlike cryotherapy chambers, they are designed to be open at the top, leaving the participant's head out, therefore removing the feeling of claustrophobia. This treatment is also called whole-body cryotherapy.

Although liquid nitrogen is used to create the cold temperature, your body is never in direct contact with the gas. As the skin responds to the cold, it sends signals to the brain. These signals revitalize the body, boosting areas that might not be functioning to their fullest potential—this process is known as vasoconstriction.

Vasoconstriction occurs when there is a narrowing of blood vessels and toxins are expelled from the outer tissue. As the body warms up again, blood that is filled with nutrients, oxygen, and enzymes flows back into the blood vessels in a process called vasodilation. As a result, the body starts all its automatic healing capabilities and releases endorphins for further well-being. Whole-body cryotherapy is very beneficial for athletic healing and muscle restoration, reducing chronic pain and inflammation. It also aids in general health and wellness[1].

Cryotherapy chambers offer the same benefits as cryo saunas, except you step into it as if you're stepping into a small room. Those who experience claustrophobia may not enjoy the closed space.

Full-body cryotherapy requires exposing your body to an extremely cold environment of -220 °F (-105 °C) and less. This acute cooling causes a number of physiologic changes in your body. During cold exposure, blood rushes away from your extremities to surround your vital organs, forcing your heart to pump more efficiently. Blood, rich with oxygen, pumps through all your vessels to supply every part of your body with the nutrients it needs. This practice, when done routinely, can help improve blood circulation, leading to a healthier heart, mind, and body.

Localized units are designed to manage inflammation and swelling on the joints and muscles. The use of localized units is the most instant and the most common form of cryotherapy. We all experience small injuries in our daily lives, but not everyone can afford to visit expensive cryo chambers to suppress the inflammation. In these instances, localized methods are the best options for small and medium injuries.

Cryo facial machines

It may not seem like a great idea to freeze your face, but that's precisely what a cryotherapy facial does. Many people, including celebrities like Jennifer Aniston, are firm believers in this method for rejuvenating their skin for a younger look without resorting to Botox injections or surgery. That's why it is playfully referred to as "frotox."

A cryotherapy facial machine uses either liquid nitrogen (also known as dry ice) or an electric heat exchange mechanism.

A cryo facial is a pleasant experience and will include the following procedures:

- You will need to remove any jewelry.
- Your face will be cleansed.
- Some practitioners will steam your face, while

others may opt to gently massage your face to promote lymphatic drainage.

- You will be given goggles to protect your eyes.
- Next, the practitioner will gently blow liquid nitrogen all over your face. You can opt to have your neck done too.
- A cryotherapy facial session lasts between three to five minutes.
- After the procedure, your skin will feel tighter and smoother.
- Once the session is over, your protective goggles are removed, and the practitioner will apply moisturizer or serum, possibly followed by a face massage.

What are the risks and side effects of cryotherapy facials?

Although they are considered safe, there are some precautions and a few reported side effects.

- Use the liquid nitrogen machine in a well-ventilated room. Nitrogen can cause an oxygen deficiency in a small, airtight space.
- The vapor is extremely cold, ranging in temperature from -200°F (-129°C) to -300°F (-184°C). In rare cases, ice burn or frostbite have been reported.

- You may experience temporary numbness or tingling. The same as if you held your hand under ice water.
- Some people have reported skin discoloration. The risk of discoloration is more common in people with darker skin tones.

What are the benefits of cryotherapy facials?

The intense cold causes your pores to tighten and blood vessels to contract. As your skin returns to its normal temperature, the blood vessels expand again quickly. This causes an increase in the flow of blood, rich in oxygen, to the face. Your skin is left looking vibrant.

Other benefits of cryo facials include tightening pores and possibly reducing the appearance of fine lines and age spots. Some studies suggest that facial cryotherapy can reduce sebum production, thereby reducing acne, but more research is needed.

At present, the most common facial cryotherapy apparatus uses liquid nitrogen. However, there is an increasing interest in electric cryotherapy. Let's have a look at the pros and cons of nitrogen-based cryo facial machines and 100% electric cryo facial machines.

Nitrogen-based cryo facial machine

Pros

• Can reach temperatures between -200°F (-129°C) and -300°F (-184°C).

Cons

• It is costly – the standard retail price was $14, 000 at the time of writing this book.

• Reoccurring cost of nitrogen.

100% Electric Cryo Facial Machine

Pros

• The standard retail price is $7, 000. Half the price of the nitrogen-based machine.

• No reoccurring nitrogen costs.

• Offers the same beauty and health benefits as nitrogen-based models.

Cons

• Some reports say that the electric cryo facial machines don't get as cold as the nitrogen-based models.

At the time of writing this book, cryotherapy treatments ranged from $20 to $200 per session, depending on the type of machine and the level of treatment. Be sure to use a trusted clinic if you'd like to try any cryotherapy treatments.

Cryotherapy treatment is not for everyone. Personally, I prefer the cold plunge. However, due to increased awareness, the cryotherapy market is growing.

According to a report by Polaris Market Research, the global cryotherapy market size was estimated at $3.51 billion in 2019 and is anticipated to grow at a rate of 9.8% from 2020-2026.[2]

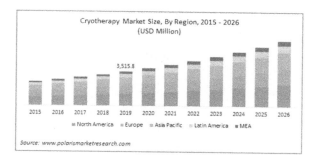

A rise in the cryotherapy market is being driven by various factors, such as the increasing number of sports injuries, skin cancers, and technological developments in cryotherapy technology.

MARKET FORCES

Driver: Technological development in cryotherapy appliances

Cryotherapy has become a popular treatment choice, largely due to the different technological innovations and developments in cryotherapy appliances over the years. Advancements have been seen in several appliances, including cryosurgery units and attachments. Cryo chambers and cryo saunas, which are used to treat pain management, rheumatoid arthritis, and inflammation, along with wellness and beauty therapies, have also experienced developmental advancements.

Furthermore, cryosurgical equipment has seen notable advancements, such as the utilization of supercooled liquid nitrogen or other cryogens for cooling, the establishment of slim and coherent probes which are available in different sizes, and the use of thin and enhanced cryoablation needles.

Vital market players

The major sellers in the cryotherapy market are: CooperSurgical (US), Galil Medical (US), and Medtronic (Ireland). These big players provide a wide product selection and have market share globally. Other sellers in this market are: Erbe Elektromedizin (Germany),

CryoConcepts (US), Impact Cryotherapy (US), Professional Products (US), Zimmer MedizinSysteme (Germany), Metrum Cryoflex (Poland), Brymill Cryogenic Systems (UK), Kriosystem Life (Poland), and US Cryotherapy (US).

I'm not here to advise you on which company is best. You will need to do your research and due diligence before purchasing.

Should you consider buying a used cryo machine?

If you're in the market for a used machine, find out its current worth, ascertain its condition, and what type of repairs (if any) it needs. Also, learn a bit about the seller to determine whether or not you should buy from them.

Nowadays, finding new and used cryo machines of all shapes, sizes, and budget ranges is easier thanks to the internet. You can simply browse online; a quick google search will reveal what is available near you.

Some celebrities love whole-body cryotherapy so much that they've set up their very own cryo chambers in their homes. Here are some celebrities that swear by cryotherapy:

- Daniel Craig
- Jennifer Aniston

- Floyd Mayweather
- Lebron James
- Usain Bolt
- Hugh Jackman
- Kevin Hart
- Cristiano Ronaldo
- Jessica Alba
- Shaquille O'Neal
- Michael Phelps
- Conor McGregor
- Novak Djokovic
- Tony Robbins
- Teemu Selänne
- Katy Perry

I hope you know by now, however, that you certainly don't need to be a celebrity to enjoy the benefits of cryotherapy.

Cryotherapy has been used for decades in cryoablation and cryosurgery, where extremely cold substances, like liquid nitrogen, are used to destroy diseased skin cells or tissue. In more acute cases, cryotherapy is used in localized treatment whenever we put an ice pack on a minor injury. Just think of all the times people have reached for the frozen peas to treat a black eye, bee sting, minor burn, or strained muscle.

Other forms of localized Cryotherapy

Ice massage

An ice massage is beneficial for localized problems like pain, swelling, and inflammation that can be caused by any number of things, including sports injury or conditions like arthritis. Ice massage is a form of cryotherapy that requires gentle pressure on the affected area with a block of ice. You can use an ice cube, but I found that it's easier to use an 'ice cup.'

To make an ice cup, simply freeze water in a small foam cup. Once the water is frozen, peel back about half an inch of foam to expose the ice. The remaining foam makes it easier for you to hold onto the ice. As the ice melts down, you can peel away more of the cup.

Avoid rubbing the ice over boney areas like your ankle, knee, elbow, shoulder blade, and spine. Gently rub the ice in small circles over the affected area.

Ice packs

As opposed to ice massage, the ice is held on the injured spot instead of being rubbed over it. You can use any pliable container to hold the ice. For example, a dish towel, plastic bag, or a commercially made ice pack. Hold the ice pack in place for up to 10 minutes. Wait at least 45 minutes before icing again.

Gel packs

Gel packs are localized units that offer quick pain relief. The gel is a mixture that does not freeze, so although it is really cold, it is still pliable. Gel packs are a successful alternative to ice packs and ice bags. The only difference between ice packs and gels packs is that the latter molds well to fit the affected body parts.

Gel packs can be conveniently kept in a freezer until they are needed. Some packs contain small gel beads made from sodium polyacrylate, which can be harmful if swallowed. Others are filled with water, silica gel, a thickening agent, a chemical to reduce the freezing temperature, and blue coloring. Whatever you do, do not ingest the gel.

Chemical cold bags

These bags are commercially manufactured localized units that become colder when the bag is squeezed. The bags are packed with water and a chemical reactor. When the bag is compressed, the water mixes with the reactor, resulting in a reaction that reduces the temperature of the water to nearly freezing. The chemical reactors in these ice packs are normally ammonium nitrate, calcium, or urea. They can be stored for long periods of time at room temperature.

Cold compression

Cold compression, although a type of cryotherapy, is also known as hilotherapy. It is generally used to treat inflammation and pain after acute injury or surgery.

The main reason for using cold compression is to accelerate outer pressure on the tissue to avoid swelling, preventing fluid loss from the vessels at the point of injury. Ice accompanied by compression is colder than ice alone due to better skin contact caused by prolonged static compression. The tissue reaches its lowest temperature more rapidly and stays cold for longer even after the treatment ends.

Many of the ice wraps available for this purpose have adjustable elastic bands which aid in the compression over the injury. More advanced individual-use wraps have instructions that specify how the band should be applied to attain optimal compression.

Most ice bandages have a built-in defensive layer so that the ice does not come into direct contact with the skin, which may result in a condition known as a cryoburn.

Whirlpool

A whirlpool is a tub filled with freezing water. Some are just big enough for an arm or a leg; others are big enough for a whole body. The body part that needs treatment is placed in the water. A small motor agitates the water so that it circulates around the injured limb.

Whirlpools can be used to decrease swelling, control inflammation, promote wound healing, improve motion, decrease pain, and decrease muscle spasms.

The water in a whirlpool can be hot or cold. Warm whirlpools increase circulation. The average temperature of a warm whirlpool is between 98°F (36°C) and 110°F (43°C).

Cold whirlpools help decrease circulation to the part of the body that is being treated. This helps in the management of inflammation and swelling. The average temperature of a cold whirlpool is generally between 50°F (10°C) and 60°F (15°C).

Important note: *Cryotherapy is not suitable for everyone. Cryo healthcare states that it should not be used by pregnant women or people with health conditions, including acute hypertension and heart problems. Anyone under 18 years of age needs parental consent.*

NATURAL DEEP-FREEZING COLD EXPOSURE

Some people prefer more natural ways of practicing cryotherapy that does not involve owning or visiting a cryotherapy sauna or chamber. Cold lakes or pools or snowy areas are places where experienced people can take their cold exposure to another level.

Please, be wise.

- Don't get into a lake that is covered in ice.

- Don't get into a river that has a strong current.

- Don't go too far into the ocean.

- Don't attempt any outdoor cold exposure practices on your own.

To up your cold exposure game, you could:

- Climb into a pond, lake, or the sea when the air and water temperature is below 40 °F (4.4°C) and take a dip.
- Go trekking/running wearing a minimum amount of clothing when the air temperature is below 40°F (4.4°C).
- Go for a stroll in the snow wearing minimal clothing.

The advantage I find with entering a cold lake or the sea compared with a shower is that you don't have that hot water setting to fall back on (which can be so tempting). Once you are in, you are totally committed.

The benefits of swimming in ice-cold water are the same as dunking yourself in an ice bath, with the added excitement of being outdoors and in nature.

Apart from boosting your immune system, improving circulation, reducing stress, and easing sore or inflamed muscles, swimming in a cold lake, ocean or river burns more calories than sitting in an ice bath, and it will leave you feeling exhilarated.

Listen to your body. Know your limits. Don't go from splashing your face with cold water to full immersion in two days and expect to stay in the water for ten minutes. Always start slowly and only attempt full immersion in a controlled setting first.

Wim Hof may have swum under a sheet of ice for more than fifty meters, but he had been practicing cold exposure for many, many years before he attempted it, and he was surrounded by a support crew.

Note: Outdoor cold exposure is not to be taken lightly. Treat the cold with respect.

GET COMFORTABLE BEING UNCOMFORTABLE

"What doesn't kill you makes you stronger." — *Friedrich Nietzsche - German philosopher*

GOOD STRESS VERSUS BAD STRESS

I'm sure you've heard many times that stress is bad for us and we should avoid it at all costs. However, not all stress is equal. There is such a thing as good stress. Referred to as eustress, good stress is beneficial and can make us feel alive and excited about our lives. It can increase our productivity and creativity and promote growth.

Has there been a time in your life that you felt stressed as you strived to meet a deadline or to make an important decision? The stress you felt would have pushed you to operate at a higher level and ultimately allow you to grow as an individual.

As humans, we all experience mental and/or physical stress; both can be acute or chronic. Acute stress, like the example of meeting a work deadline, can help us improve our level of alertness and behavioral and cognitive performance. Similarly, working out is a form of stressing the body physically. Again, the stress caused by working out allows the body to adapt and to grow during the recovery phase, leaving us in a better place than when we started.

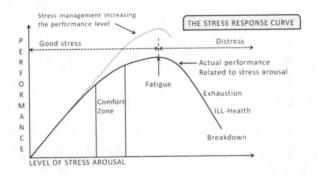

Human response to stress curve (*according to Nixon P: Practitioner 1979, Yerkes RM, Dodson JD). [1]

The type of stress that we should do our best to avoid is chronic stress. Whereas acute stress can raise us to new heights, chronic stress can have many negative effects on your emotional and physical health. It can manifest in feelings of overwhelm, irritability, fatigue, and even depression.

Your perception is a very important tool in your arsenal when protecting against stress. The exact same situation can be perceived by two people in completely different ways. If you feel that a stressful situation is something that you can overcome, then the stress you experience will be reduced. If you feel that the situation is outside of your capacity, then the feelings of stress are likely to be higher. Another important note here is remembering to 'control the controllable.' It's futile to stress over something that is outside of your control.

Stanford Psychologist Kelly McGonigal, in her 2013 TED talk 'How to make stress your friend,'[2] claims that it is not stress that kills you; it's the story you tell yourself about stress.

McGonigal administered a socially evaluated stress test to teach participants how to improve their stress response. She concluded that participants who were told that their stress responses were *helpful* experienced an elevated heart rate, which is a typical stress response. However, they didn't experience the usual constriction of blood vessels—the thing that makes stress bad for our hearts. We may not be able to rid our lives of stress, but we can learn to interpret it differently so that it's not as harmful.

Cold exposure is a way of intentionally inducing stress, but in a controlled manner. When stress is mild and controllable, it can lead to positive outcomes later in life. The reason for repeatedly inducing short bouts of physical stress is for the body and brain to adapt to accommodate stress. After making cold exposure a habit, you will be able to control the stress of the cold. Cold exposure teaches us that we can control our stress response. Initially, cold water will induce a cold shock response, which is a gasp reflex—rapid breathing that subsides as your body becomes accustomed to the cold temperature. The more often you are exposed to the cold, the more accustomed you will be to the shock response.

One way psychologists evaluate stress response is by using a Socially Evaluated Cold Pressor Test[3] (SECPT). The test involves subjects immersing one hand in cold water for three minutes. The test generates a strong response from the sympathetic nervous system. Subjects heart rate and blood pressure increase, stress hormones cortisol and norepinephrine increase. Essentially the body goes into fight or flight mode, which is the body's natural response to danger.

A 2014 study[4] showed that the physiological effects of cold stress are reduced over repeated exposures. Heart rate response to SECPT was less during the third exposure compared to the first. Subjects' perceptions of the stress and cortisol release were also reduced upon repeat exposure. These findings suggest that the body's physiological and psychological responses to stress can be trained. Wim Hoff has completed some amazing feats like running a half marathon at the Arctic Circle barefoot, swimming under the ice for 66 meters, and climbing the highest mountains in the world wearing only shorts. Wim Hof also managed to stay submerged in an ice bath for 112 minutes without his core body temperature changing. He is only able to achieve this because he has conditioned his body and mind to cope with these stresses through repeated exposure. Therefore, to improve our stress response and maybe our performance under pressure, we need to *practice experiencing stress*. If you can cope with the savage nature of the cold, you can cope with anything.

THE BATTLE IS WON IN YOUR MIND

How we think touches every aspect of our lives, from how we understand purpose, value, and meaning, to our ability to master new skills and adopt positive life changes.

Despite the constant changes in our external environment, the real battle is within - real change can't happen until we change our minds and our thoughts.

Our thoughts – and the power they have to change our minds – play a vital role in how we experience our reality and shape our future.

Our brains seek patterns to aid our survival. If we can fall back on a familiar pattern, it doesn't take too much energy to face situations similar to anything we've faced before. This pattern-seeking develops actions that become habits.

In the same way we develop habits of action concerning our environment, we develop habits of thought. One of the reasons we find it so hard to change our minds is because our brains are stuck in this circular rut that always has us looking at things from one perspective – our own past experiences.

We have the power and ability to break our minds out of the rut, but first, we must realize there is a necessity to do just that.

Changing our thinking changes us

Everyone thinks differently based on their unique upbringing and biology. In order for two people to think the same, they would have had to live exactly the same life. It's interesting to note that it is our thinking patterns that make us who we are. The wider the scope of our thoughts, the better we will be able to interact with what is going on around us.

This would explain terms such as 'open-minded' instead of 'narrow-minded.' I had to broaden my thinking when I decided to investigate cold exposure. I had to change my mind about loving the feeling of cold water on my body instead of hot. I had to adopt a new mindset about climbing into a tub or lake of icy water. My body couldn't do any of those things until I'd made up my mind that I needed to.

"The greatest discovery of my generation is that a human being can alter his life by altering his attitudes of mind." — William James

Throughout our life experiences, we begin to develop thought patterns and absorb them as part of our reality. We learn about what things we like (e.g., warm water) and what situations cause us discomfort or pain (e.g., cold water). Our brain forms habits of action and habits of thought around these stimuli.

The downside is that it is so easy for us to get stuck in a mental rut which is often limiting when the situation requires us to think 'out of the box.' To overcome this, we must purposefully change our thinking patterns to be able to make new connections between our thoughts and the world around us.

Startling truth:

How we process what is happening to us is more important than what is happening to us.

Once you've overcome the battle in your mind, you're more than halfway to developing a habit of daily cold showers and regular full-body cold therapy.

PRACTICAL STEPS TO HELP YOU GET STARTED

For most of us, the advantages of cold immersion begin at any temperature that makes us uneasy yet still enables us to make the practice part of our routine. As you become more accustomed to the practice, you can lower the water temperature and/or extend the amount of time you remain submersed.

Here are a few practical tips that will make the journey from a quick cold shower to a full-body immersion in icy water a lot more enjoyable and, therefore, highly more likely to end in success:

1. Have a dry towel and clothes close by.

This is where the 'easing in gently' concept will come into play. Your body will be feeling really chilly after your cold exposure. Having a dry towel and clothes close by will be a reward you can look forward to after a cold shower. Their close proximity will escalate to an absolute necessity once you begin extreme full-body exposure, especially if you're outdoors in winter.

2. Dip your hands and feet in the cold water first.

Whether it's your first cold shower or your first full body plunge, put your hands and feet in the water first. This will only be necessary in the beginning. Once you've practiced cold exposure a few times, this step will not be necessary.

3. Splash cold water onto your body.

Once again, this is something you will only have to do at the beginning of your cold exposure journey. Using cupped hands, splash some water onto a dry area of your body, such as your face, head, legs, arms, or torso.

You can repeat this process until you've wet your entire body. This will help your body to prepare for going under the cold water.

4. Listen to music to help you stay calm and focused.

Music has always been one of our greatest allies when it comes to overcoming negative emotions. If you find you are tense or fearful in the beginning, you can play calming music or your favorite upbeat music to help.

The goal is to distract yourself from the short-term discomfort and push forward. You could create a playlist of two or three songs. This will be beneficial because you can use the songs as a timer as well. After the first song, you know you've been in the water for, say, two and a half minutes. This will help you to stop clock-watching and enable you to enjoy the moment more.

5. Let your brain tell your body that you enjoy cold exposure.

As I explained earlier in the book, the attitude of your mind has a huge impact on whether or not new experiences are conceived as positive or negative. Your internal dialogue can be a major source of inspiration and motivation, or it can kill the experience—you decide. Give yourself a motivational talk before getting into the cold water.

Some positive affirmation you can think or say include:

- I love how energized cold exposure leaves me feeling.
- I can feel my body responding positively to the cold.
- Cold exposure is great for my body and mind.
- I'm unstoppable after cold exposure.
- My day goes from good to great after cold exposure.
- If I can stand cold exposure, I can deal with anything life throws my way.
- My cold exposure routine proves how disciplined I am.
- This is making me healthier.

While I was still adapting to the cold water, my favorite saying was, "This too shall pass!"

It's amazing what positive self-talk can do to enhance your attitude.

6. **Focus on your breathing.**

Wim Hof himself says that cold exposure is not only about the cold but also about breathing and commitment—it's a triangle of discipline.

Your breath is a monitor for your nervous system. You can excite yourself by breathing faster and shallowly or calm yourself by breathing slower and deeper.

Being able to control your breathing is an important way to manage your physical and mental health. Monks are known to meditate under cold waterfalls and control their breathing to produce heat in their bodies to combat the extremely cold temperatures. You can use your breathing in a similar way during cold exposure.

Concentrate on your breathing and *feel* how it changes when you step into the cold shower. Usually, the cold water will make you take fast, shallow breaths at first. Concentrate on deep, slow breaths. If you can control your breathing, you'll be amazed by how much more power you have in any given situation.

7. <u>Visualize you're somewhere beautiful to help relax yourself.</u>

If you're taking a cold shower, imagining you're standing under a pristine waterfall in a beautiful mountainous setting may help. If you're immersed in a tub of icy water, picturing yourself in a lake or river in a green forest may be all the distraction you need to help you stay under the water for a few minutes.

8. Ease in.

To begin with, you don't have to jump into an ice-cold shower immediately. It's easier to begin with lukewarm water and then slowly work your way to colder temperatures as your body adjusts.

If you put a frog in hot water, it will jump out. However, if you raise the temperature slowly, the frog will not realize it until the water is boiling and it's too late. To the opposite degree but not nearly as extreme, if you lower the shower water temperature gradually or adjust the temperature of the ice tub water slowly over time, your body will acclimate, and you're more likely to persevere than if you shock yourself into not enjoying the experience.

Always give yourself a fair chance, or you may avoid the situation completely.

Contrast showers

Another way of easing in is to take contrast showers. This means switching between hot and cold temperatures.

- Use 45 seconds cold and 15 seconds hot ratio, or any other that makes you more likely to follow through with your cold showers.
- Using heat for a few seconds will give your

muscles a few seconds to relax and, in turn, let your skin temperature warm up.

- Once you switch back to cold water, you will feel a little recharge and shake off any discomfort again.

Keep in mind when taking contrast showers that you should end the shower at a cold temperature to reap all the benefits.

9. Turn it into a game or a challenge.

It's human nature to be competitive, most of us enjoy a challenge. If you challenge someone or if you are challenged it usually leads to an attitude of "No matter what, I need to do this!"

Turn your cold exposure into a personal challenge.

Set a timer before every session and see how long you last. Make sure that you record your score every day and track your progress. This can be a truly fun way to force yourself to go that extra mile. Make it your target to smash your high score every week or month.

Important Note:

Turning cold therapy into a competition against other people is not a great idea. Everyone responds differently to cold exposure. In a competitive environment, people may be inclined to ignore the warning signs that they have reached their limit, which could lead to risky behavior that can endanger health and wellbeing. In all your challenges, you should only be competing against yourself—and even then, proceed with caution.

10. <u>Pretend you're a hero.</u>

If all you need is a little distraction to help you bide the time while you stand under or plunge into cold water, you could visualize yourself as a hero in an action movie. Imagine that you're working your way through rugged terrain to kill a dragon or pretend you're a survivor in the arctic attempting to find warmth, shelter, and food.

If you can tap into your imagination, you can gain extra inspiration and motivation that you didn't realize you had. We often give up this power of visualization as we get older, but it's an ability we should practice throughout our lives.

THE 30-DAY COLD SHOWER CHALLENGE

Corresponding with the techniques I described above, you can take the 30-day cold shower challenge. Based on my experience of coaching beginners on cold immersion, I recommend progressing through your 30-day challenge in three phases.

Phase 1 (Day 1-10): Start end each day by taking a 60-second cold shower. No days off. This can be achieved in different ways, but my two favorites are:

- One-minute straight. Take a one-minute cold shower at the end of your normal shower. Remember to take long, deep breaths the entire time to calm your nervous system.
- "Tabata" cold showering: Stand under cold water for 20 seconds and then under hot water for 10. Repeat eight times. Another way of doing this is to stand under the cold water for 20 seconds and then step out from under the water for 10, rather than adjusting the water temperature. You can use a timing app to help you track the intervals.

Remember that the first two to three days are the hardest when you start your cold shower routine. Ease yourself in gently but motivate yourself to stick with it by thinking of the health and wellness benefits that cold exposure brings. After three days, you will already start to feel amazing.

Phase 2 (Day 11-20): Start every day with a two- to three-minute cold shower after your regular shower. Take days 14 and 20 off. If you choose the Tabata method, extend the time that you spend under cold water.

Phase 3 (Day 21-30): Start every day with a five-minute cold shower after your regular shower. Take days 24 and 28 off. By now, your body will have become more accustomed to the cold water, and the benefits will be outweighing the discomfort at this stage.

If you've made it this far and enjoy feeling invigorated every day, you are ready to take on a complete cold shower from start to finish. Like the classic Nike slogan suggests - Just do it!

NATURE HAS IT ALL

People who live in cold areas and want to practice cold exposure are at an advantage. You can choose ponds, pools, and lakes for your extreme cold exposure sessions. If you live in a cold area, try some of the following cold exposure experiences:

- Go for a brief swim wearing only swimwear in a pond or lake where the water temperature is below 40° F (5° C).
- If you live in hilly areas, go trekking or running wearing a minimal amount of clothes when the air temperature is below 40° F (5° C).

- If there is snowfall in your area, go for a barefoot stroll in the snow or try to sit or lie down in the snow for a few minutes at a time.

"The magic is doing the simple things repeatedly and long enough to ignite the miracle of the compound effect." — *Darren Hardy*

A NOTE ON HYPOTHERMIA

I started this chapter with the quote, *"What doesn't kill you makes you stronger,"* and there is hardly a truer warning when it comes to cold exposure and hypothermia. I wrote this book to tell you about the benefits of cold exposure and how practicing it can make you stronger – but you need to be aware that extreme cold can kill you.

Hypothermia occurs when the body's core temperature drops below 98.6° F (35°C). Regardless of whether the external conditions are warm or cold, our bodies are conditioned to keep our core temperate consistent. If the body's core temperate drops just 2 or 3 degrees below 98.6° F, we go into a hypothermic state. When your temperature drops even further, the state can be irreversible and will continue to drop. Hypothermia is a medical emergency and, if not treated, will cause your vital organs to shut down, resulting in death.

Signs and symptoms of hypothermia:

- Shivering
- Slurred speech
- Slow, shallow breathing
- Weak pulse
- Lack of coordination
- Drowsiness
- Confusion
- Loss of consciousness
- Bright red, cold skin

It is imperative that if you are engaging in cold therapy (especially outside in nature) that you DO NOT do it alone. People with hypothermia aren't usually aware of it in the beginning because the symptoms often develop gradually. The confusion that comes with hypothermia can prevent self-awareness. Pay attention to your body and, when you are practicing cold exposure with others, keep checking in on them.

6

FORMING A NEW HABIT

"In essence, if we want to direct our lives, we must take control of our consistent actions. It's not what we do once in a while that shapes our lives, but what we do consistently." — *Tony Robbins*

A SMALL CHANGE IN HABITS MAKES A HUGE DIFFERENCE

It is so easy to underestimate the value of making tiny improvements on a day-to-day basis. Too often, we persuade ourselves that great success requires massive deeds. Whether it is mastering cold exposure, writing a book, losing weight, winning a championship, building a business, or achieving any other target, we pressure ourselves to make an out-of-this-world improvement that everyone will speak about.

Statistically, improving by 1% isn't especially noteworthy – sometimes, it isn't even detectable. However, a 1% improvement, consistently and over the long-term, can be very significant. Tiny consistent improvements lead to outstanding results.

Mathematically speaking, good habits are the compound interest of self-improvement. These habits don't make much difference on any particular day, yet their impact over the months and years that follow can be immeasurable.

The compound effect can be a difficult concept to grasp in everyday life. We frequently ignore small changes because they don't appear to matter very much in a particular moment. If you save a little money for a few months, you won't become a millionaire. If you go to the gym three days in a row, you'll still be out of shape. If you study Italian for an hour, you won't master the language. Although changes have been set in motion, the outcomes do not appear instantly, so we are at risk of reverting back to our former routines.

Unfortunately, because of this principle, it's easy to allow bad habits to stick. If you consume an unhealthy meal today, the scales won't move much tomorrow. If you work late tonight and take no notice of your family, they will pardon you. A single unhealthy act is easy to overlook.

However, when we repeat bad choices, night and day, replicating tiny mistakes and justifying them with excuses, the small actions accumulate into harmful results in the long run. It is an accumulation of many small missteps that finally leads to a big problem.

A negative change in your habits can be likened to changing the route of a flight by a few degrees. Assume you are flying from Los Angeles to New York City. If a pilot leaves from Los Angeles and alters the heading just 3.5 degrees south, you will land in Washington, D.C., rather than your original destination. Such a tiny change is hardly noticeable during takeoff – after all, the front of the airplane shifts just a few degrees – but in the end, you will land up hundreds of miles off course.

Similarly, a tiny positive change in your day-to-day habits can take your life to a very different level. Making a choice that is 1% beneficial or 1% harmful seems unimportant, but, over time, it makes a huge difference. These choices decide who you are and who you could be. Success is, therefore, the outcome of everyday habits.

Habit stacking

A significant amount of evidence[1] suggests that our brains are malleable and can change according to our experiences. The term *neuroplasticity* infers that our brains are not as set in their ways as we think. On the contrary, if we participate in voluntary frequent, positive, and challenging experiences, our brains begin to rewire themselves, creating new neural pathways. These new neural pathways mean we can learn new habits and unlearn old ones.

For example, if you practice cold exposure often, your brain will develop a new pathway that bypasses the 'gasp reflex.' The more you practice cold exposure, the stronger and more efficient the neural pathway will become. As your brain uses the new pathways more often, you will find it easier to push your cold exposure limits.

Let's discuss how neuroplasticity plays a vital role in forming new habits.

Your brain has built a powerful network of neurons over the years to assist you with your present behaviors. The more you do something, the deeper the neural pathway runs. Learning new things, and developing new habits, takes a bit longer, but only until the neural pathway has been established then it becomes an automatic behavior.

Let's use learning to drive as an example. There is a lot to remember when you get behind the wheel the first time. In the beginning, every move you make is deliberate and calculated, and possibly even stressful. Once you have practiced a few hours a day for a month, most of your actions are automatic and, after a year, you can drive without even thinking about it. Why? Because your brain created neural pathways, your body will automatically know how to behave when you need to drive.

You have hundreds of very powerful connections that help you do everything you need to do every day. For example, you are efficient at opening the curtains when the sun rises, brushing your teeth, getting dressed, and eating breakfast. Why? Because you've done those things every day since you can remember. The good news is that you can take advantage of the development of new neural pathways to start and maintain new good habits, like taking a cold shower each morning.

To build new habits, you can use the connectivity of behavior to your advantage. One of the best ways to build a new habit is to recognize a present habit and then stack your new habit on top of it. This is known as habit stacking.

Instead of pairing your new behavior with a definite time and location, pair it with a present habit.

For example:

After I complete my morning workout, I will stretch for 10 minutes.

After I get into bed at night, I will say one thing that I'm grateful for.

After I brush my teeth, I will take a cold shower.

One of the reasons habit stacking works so well is that your present habits already have well-established neural pathways. Pairing a new habit with an existing pathway will make it easier for you to persist.

Once you have mastered the art of stacking a new habit to an existing habit, you can make larger stacks by pairing other small habits together. This allows you to take advantage of the natural momentum that occurs from one habit and leads to the next.

Habits shape your identity

Why is it so easy to repeat bad habits yet so hard to continue with the good ones? Because *maintaining* your existing habits is easier than *cultivating* new ones – the pathways have been established, there's no 'work' involved. It's like driving on an existing road compared to forging a new one through a jungle. Unless you have the commitment to establish a new habit, this time next year, you'll be doing the same things you've always done.

It's hard to keep good behaviors going for more than a few days or weeks, even with profound effort and sporadic bursts of inspiration. New habits, like exercise, meditation, and journaling, are fun and exciting in the first few days or weeks but can sometimes become a hassle, especially when our busy lives get in the way.

Behavior that is incompatible with oneself will not last long. For example, you may desire to become rich, but if your personality favors spending over saving, then, in all probability, you'll squander rather than accumulate money. In the same way, you may wish to attain better health, but if you continue to favor comfort over achievement, you'll likely fail.

Remember, it's difficult to change your habits if you never alter the underlying programming that guided your past behavior. You may have a new objective and a new plan, but you also need to change who you are.

The final form of inherent motivation is when a habit or behavior becomes part of your identity. It's one thing to say, I'm the kind of person who *desires* this, and another to say, I'm the kind of person who *is* this.

The more fixed you are to a particular part of your identity, the more motivated you will be to keep up the habits related to it. For example, if you're proud of how your hair looks, you'll create all types of habits to care for and maintain it.

How to get out of your comfort zone

The comfort zone can keep you doing the same things year after year, getting the same results, and never improving. This comfort zone has become your identity.

New identities need new authentication. If you continue casting the same vote you've always cast, you're going to obtain the same results you've always had.

Getting out of your comfort zone, however, is an easy two-phase process:

1. Determine the kind of person you want to be.
2. Become that person with small victories.

Your habits *make a difference*. They help you become the person you desire to be. Unfortunately, they also keep you from becoming the person you desire to be. They are the path through which you build your deepest beliefs about yourself. Quite literally, *you become your habits.*

At this point, you are hopefully well aware of the importance of new behaviors in your life. Now, it's time to learn how new habits can change your routine and, ultimately, your identity.

You can change your behavior by adding cold exposure to your daily habits. You can change your true identity by practicing cold exposure repeatedly.

How to incorporate cold exposure into your new identity

Psychologist Edward Thorndike once conducted a classic experiment in which he used a puzzle box to observe habit-building in animals[2]. The box was made in such a way that a cat could get out of the box through a door by completing a simple action, such as stepping on a platform, pushing a lever, or pulling at a loop of cord.

We know that cats love boxes, but in this experiment, the cat wanted to escape as soon as it was placed inside the box because Thorndike put a piece of fish on the outside of the box. At first, the cat would nudge its nose into the corners, shove its paws through openings, and pounce at loose objects. After a few minutes of activity, the cat would escape.

As soon as the cat escaped, it was placed back into the box. In back-to-back trials, the cat learned that pushing the lever opened the door. The animal caught on to this behavior and became progressively faster at pushing the lever. After 25-30 trials, the behavior became so automatic that the cat escaped within a few seconds.

Edward Thorndike put forward a "Law of effect," which stated that any behavior that is followed by pleasant consequences is likely to be repeated, and any behavior followed by unpleasant consequences is likely to be stopped.

I have made cold exposure a habit in my life because of the way it makes me feel alive and energized. This good feeling is the pleasant outcome that reinforces the habit. If I felt awful every time I stepped out of the shower or plunge pool, I very much doubt I would have stuck with it.

According to James Clear, author of the best-selling book Atomic Habits, the Habit Loop is divided into four phases:

1) cue
2) craving

3) response
4) reward.

The cue is the first sign that we're close to getting a reward. It naturally leads to a craving. A cue can be a number of different things; time, location, a preceding event, an emotional state, or another person. You can try out these different cues and see what works best for you. I used a combination of cues to develop the habit of using the plunge pool daily.

Consider this statement: After I put a pot of coffee on to brew first thing in the morning, I take a 3-minute cold plunge outside in the garden.

There are three cues at play here: time, location, and preceding event.

1) The habit occurs at the same time every morning – as soon as I wake up.
2) The habit occurs in the same location – the garden.
3) The habit is always preceded by an event – me brewing coffee.

I chose to stack the habit of using the plunge pool on top of an already ingrained habit of brewing coffee. The other reason is that once I'm all dried off, I can enjoy a nice warm cup of coffee.

Secondly, there are the cravings. These are the influential force behind every habit or behavior. Without a craving, a habit is unlikely to last. What you crave is not the habit itself but rather the reward that comes with the habit. I don't crave jumping into the cold water, but I crave the feeling of the endorphins getting released into my bloodstream.

The response is the action you carry out that leads to the reward.

Rewards close the habit loop by satisfying your cravings. Your brain remembers which actions produce pleasurable rewards and, in the future, looks out for the cue that initiated it in the first place.

After repeating cold exposure several times and experiencing the eternal calmness it gives you physically and mentally, you will have mastered the habit of cold exposure. Each time you are exposed to the cold, you cast a vote for the person you are becoming and ultimately forging your new identity.

If a behavior is inadequate in any of the four stages, it will not become a habit. Abolish the cue, and your habit will never begin. Lessen the craving, and you won't experience enough influence to act. And, if the reward fails to please your craving, then you won't have a motive to do it again in the future. Without the first three stages, the behavior will not happen.

To sum up the habit loop: the cue incites a craving, which influences a response, which gives a reward, which pleases the craving and, ultimately, becomes a permanent habit.

THE HABIT LOOP

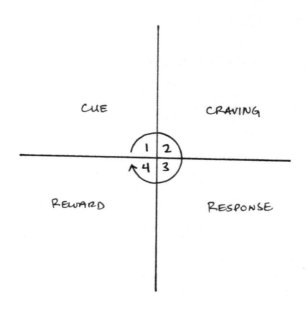

Image credit: James Clear. Atomic Habits.[3]

The habit tracker

A habit tracker is an easy way to track whether you complete a good habit. One of our challenges when it comes to adopting good habits is maintaining awareness of what we are doing. When I start any new habit, I track it on a grid on a whiteboard on my kitchen wall. I have the days of the week down one column and the habits across the top row. Once the action is completed, I simply put a tick in the box. It gives me such a sense of achievement when I see a full week of ticks against the habits I'm working on. It also has incredible power for kicking me into action if, for whatever reason, I have not completed an action by the evening. I hate seeing a blank space on that whiteboard. I don't want to break the chain. It's a simple concept but incredibly powerful. This practice can easily be replicated with a wall calendar (if you're only tracking one or two habits) where you check off the day once you have completed your habit. Keep it somewhere visible so that you can clearly see your progress. Tracking apps can be used but personally I like something that is visual and is there for everyone to see.

Set the right environment

Self-discipline is overrated when it comes to habits. Setting the right environment, however, is where the real power lies. I'm sure you've heard before that if you want to make a habit of going to the gym each morning, then laying out your running shoes and gym kit the night before significantly increases your chances of going. The last thing you want is to be scrambling around for your kit first thing in the morning. Setting out the kit reduces friction. Reduce friction, and you will be far more likely to succeed in sticking with your habits. Everyone has a slightly different home environment, but we can change our environment to best suit us. Before going to bed, I check that there is enough ice in the freezer for the plunge pool and set out a towel for the next morning. When it comes to my morning routine of cold exposure, the fewer barriers, the better.

Be accountable

Having an accountability partner is another powerful way of making sure you stick with your new habits. Going back to the early morning gym example, if you have arranged to meet your training partner at the gym at 6 am, you are far less likely to press the snooze button and go back to sleep. The thought of not letting your friend down is a greater force than the inconvenience of getting up and getting to the gym.

The way I use accountability with cold exposure is that I have a written contract with my friend. If I miss more than five days of cold exposure in a given month, I have to give him $50 at the end of that month. Lucky for me,

I am his accountability partner, so the same rules apply to him.

Sometimes the motivation to avoid pain is just as powerful as the motivation to achieve pleasure. Use something that will work for you. My motivation for avoiding pain is compounded by the opportunity to achieve pleasure. If I have had a full week of cold exposure, I reward myself with a couple of beers on a Saturday evening.

I like to think of this multi-pronged approach to motivation as tripling my chances of success:

- Some days I'm motivated purely by the benefits of cold exposure.
- Some days I'm motivated by not wanting to hand $50 to my friend.
- Other days I'm motivated by the prospect of those ice-cold beers.

"Don't break the chain. It is the key to success."

7

CONTRAST TEMPERATURE THERAPY

We've spent the last six chapters of this book exploring the ins and outs of cold therapy. Now, we're going to look at contrast temperature therapy. Why? Because, like cold therapy, it is a health and lifestyle-enhancing modality that has been practiced for many years in different cultures, but I don't believe the benefits are publicized enough.

WHAT IS CONTRAST TEMPERATURE THERAPY?

Contrast temperature therapy is the act of moving from a hot environment to a cold one, back and forth, several times with no rest period in between to allow the body to acclimate naturally.

The 'hot' environment can be a hot shower, a bath, tub, or pool filled with hot water, a natural hot spring, or a sauna. The 'cold' environment can be any of the cold exposure experiences we discussed earlier in the book; namely, a cold shower, a bath, tub, or pool filled with icy cold water, a naturally icy lake, or a cryotherapy chamber.

Contrast temperature therapy can be as simple as standing under a hot shower for a few minutes before turning the hot water off and standing under a cold shower, repeating the hot-cold exposure. Or it can be as adventurous as getting out of a sauna or hot tub and immersing yourself in an icy lake—people have been doing it for years in Scandinavian countries.

We are designed to withstand a certain range of temperature changes. When we get hot, our heart rate increases, our blood pressure goes up, our blood gets thinner, and rushes to our extremities to cool down before being pumped back to cool our core. When we get cold, our heart rate decreases, our blood pressure drops, our blood thickens, and withdraws from our extremities to keep our core warm. Both these reactions are perfectly natural.

People with certain health issues and those who are predisposed to certain conditions will want to avoid sudden and drastic changes in temperature to prevent complications. On the other hand, healthy individuals can 'force' this natural blood rush by practicing contrast therapy and, in the process, reap the health benefits.

Using a Whirlpool for contrast temperature therapy

Another way to practice contrast temperature therapy is with a Whirlpool[1] physiotherapy machine. Whirlpool therapy is a contrast bath treatment that involves using a hot whirlpool and a cold whirlpool during the same treatment.

A whirlpool is a large tub filled with either hot or cold water, depending on the physical therapy that is needed. The body part that is being treated is placed in the tub while a small motor circulates the water. During this physical therapy exercise, the body part that is being treated is moved from warm to cold water and back again every one to three minutes for a total of 15 to 20 minutes. Your physiotherapist may instruct you to move the affected limb while it is immersed in the warm water to help improve the mobility of the affected area.

Whirlpool physical therapy can be used for the following:

- Control inflammation

- Decrease swelling
- Decrease pain
- Decrease muscle spasms
- Promote wound healing
- Improve motion

When to use heat therapy versus cold therapy?

You may be wondering when to use heat to treat an injury or an ailment versus when to use cold. Briefly, heat boosts blood and nutrient flow to an area of the body, so it works well for stiffness and all related ailments. On the other hand, cold slows blood flow, reducing pain and swelling, and other related ailments.

Depending on the extent of the injury or stiffness, you can use a heat pad, hot water bottle, warm wrap, or hot water to treat ailments that require heat therapy. For ailments that respond better to cold therapy, you can use any of the methods listed in Chapter 4, where we discussed the use of localized cryotherapy in the form of ice, ice packs, or gel packs and immersion in cold water.

WHO USES CONTRAST TEMPERATURE THERAPY?

Contrast temperature therapy has been practiced in many cultures for thousands of years without being labeled as such. The Ancient Egyptians, Romans, Greeks, and Scandinavians have been using hot saunas and cold baths for health reasons for centuries. Contrast therapy has been part of ancient Chinese medicine for hundreds of years too.

Tony Robbins[2], arguably one of the most recognizable life coaches and motivational speakers in the world, starts each day with a workout followed by an extra-hot sauna and a plunge in an ice-cold pool.

People think that saunas are just there to get rid of toxins, but while that is true, that is not their only benefit. Robbins says that the contrast temperature exposure after his morning gym routine acts as an extension of the time spent working out instead of being just another ordinary spa-day activity.

Some American football teams, including the Arizona Cardinals, Cincinnati Bengals, Dallas Cowboys, Detroit Lions, Kansas City Chiefs, New York Jets, New York Giants, Philadelphia Eagles, Pittsburgh Steelers, and Tampa Bay Buccaneers, use contrast therapy treatment as part of their training and recovery routines.

A Scottish shower

A Scottish shower is a type of contrast therapy and involves a very hot shower followed by at least one minute of icy cold water. This isn't quite the same as the contrast therapy of going from hot to cold and back again several times for the duration of your shower. This protocol is the same as the beginner stage of developing the cold shower habit where you take a warm shower but finish with cold water. The health benefits of a Scottish shower include enhancing circulation, boosting your immune system, stimulating fat loss, helping you sleep better, and improving skin and hair.

Precautionary notes:

- Combining hot saunas and cold plunges can be dangerous if you have certain health conditions, are taking certain medications, or are pregnant.
- Different temperatures cause changes in how your heart beats—cold water causes your heart rate to slow down, while hot water will cause it to speed up.
- Always speak to a healthcare professional before starting a new healthcare practice.

WHAT ARE THE HEALTH BENEFITS OF CONTRAST TEMPERATURE THERAPY?

Contrast temperature therapy and arthritis

Since contrast therapy improves your blood circulation, it is helpful in the treatment of stiff joints, edema, inflammation of soft tissue, painful limbs, and muscle spasms.

Many doctors recommend both hot and cold therapy for the treatment of arthritis, pain, and stiffness. The contrast therapy can range between heating and cooling pads (dry exposure) to hot and cold showers or full immersion (wet exposure).

Contrast therapy works by using your body's natural self-healing abilities. For example, applying heat causes blood vessels to dilate, stimulates circulation, and reduces muscle spasms. Cold exposure restricts blood vessels, reduces swelling, and can ultimately numb the pain.

Contrast temperature therapy promotes general health and wellbeing

Contrast showers

"Contrast showers increase blood flow and stabilize it at the same time, perfect for rebooting your systems. This boosts your immune system, improves testosterone levels, cuts the downtime for muscle recovery after intense physical activity, and improves heart health." —Dr. Gan Eng Cern, physician, ear, nose, and throat surgeon and member of the Royal College of Surgeons at Edinburgh, United Kingdom. [3]

Both hot and cold showers benefit your body in different ways. We're inclined to favor hot showers because they make us feel more comfortable. However, adding cold showers to our daily routine brings tremendous health benefits:

- Improved concentration
- Boosted immune response
- Higher energy levels
- Increased metabolism
- Improved sleep
- Reduced inflammation, muscle soreness,

THE COLD THERAPY CODE | 133

stiffness, and swelling, as we read in the earlier chapters of this book.

Now, we're learning that contrast showers have certain benefits of their own.

The hot water opens your blood vessels and gets your blood pumping quickly. When you switch to cold water, it has the opposite effect, closing blood vessels and pushing blood back towards your internal organs. The opening and closing of blood vessels results in a push-pull of freshly oxygenated blood, promoting detoxification.

Contrast showers also help boost mitochondrial health. An increase in mitochondrial cells results in increased energy. Briefly, mitochondria use the oxygen available in the cell to convert chemical energy into useable energy. When you work out, you use your mitochondria cells—the more energy you have, the harder and longer you can work out. Contrast showers stimulate your mitochondria in a similar way due to the rapid in and outflow of oxygenated blood.

Advice for taking a contrast shower

If you are still not convinced that a cold shower is a great ritual to add to your daily routine, you'll be pleased to hear that contrast showers have health benefits too.

One way you can introduce contrast temperature exposure to your shower time is to start with a hot shower while you wash and then turn the hot water off until you are standing under a stream of cold water.

Remember not to tense up; try and keep your breathing as natural as possible. Use some of the cold exposure tips I shared with you in Chapter 5, like taking slow deep breaths, visualization, gamification, or listening to music.

Stand under the cold water for 30 seconds and then turn the hot water back on. Repeat three or four times. After a few days, try and make the cold part of the shower go on for longer. The most important thing is to end with cold water for as long as possible.

Hot and cold plunges

For those who want to participate in something a little more 'extreme' than contrast showers, there is the option to practice a more exhilarating type of cold therapy that includes hot and cold plunges. This can include alternating between a tub of hot water and one that's icy cold or jumping from a sauna into a really cold lake. The methods you use depend on your level of adventure and the resources you have available.

Some of the benefits of contrast therapy plunges include:

- Increased pulse rate and circulation.
- Stiff muscles, aches, and pains from intense workouts are reduced.
- When you immerse yourself in cold water after being in a hot environment, norepinephrine (an anti-stress hormone and neurotransmitter) and epinephrine (adrenaline) are released. The release of these hormones leaves you feeling invigorated.
- Immersing in cold water after a sauna has been found to reduce pain and improve circulation. This helps minimize the symptoms of rheumatoid arthritis.
- A cold exposure plunge improves the body's detoxification capabilities, increasing white blood cell count.
- Contrary to popular opinion, contrast temperature therapy helps improve the body's resistance to respiratory infections.
- Repeated contrast exposure can stabilize blood pressure and strengthen nerves in the autonomic nervous system.

Important note:

The benefits listed above pertain to healthy individuals. If you have a health condition or you're on medication, seek medical advice before practicing extreme contrast temperature exposure.

Contrast temperature therapy and injury

The theory behind using temperature therapy to treat injuries is that the contrasting temperatures create the rapid opening and closing of the arteries around the body part being treated. This, in turn, creates a pumping effect that helps reduce swelling around the injury.

Common conditions and injuries that can be treated with contrast therapy include:

- Stiff muscles after workout or sport activities
- Sore muscles after sport injury
- Achy joints after a workout or sports activities
- Ankle or wrist fracture
- Ankle or wrist sprain
- Plantar fasciitis
- Tennis elbow
- Lisfranc dislocation
- Achilles' tendon rupture
- Tendinitis

• Colles' and Smith's fractures

Step by step guide to using contrast temperature therapy to treat injuries:

1. Decide what method of contrast therapy you are going to use, for example, a hot water bottle and an ice compress or tubs – one with hot water and one with ice water.

2. A clock or stopwatch.

3. Follow this basic pattern when applying contrast therapy:

   - Start with one minute of cold
   - Apply three minutes of heat
   - Apply one minute of cold
   - Apply three minutes of heat
   - Apply one minute of cold
   - Apply three minutes of heat
   - End off with one minute of cold

4. Protect your skin against heat and ice burns with a thin layer of fabric or a towel.

5. If you can, increase the intensity of the hot and cold as you progress. That is, make the hot hotter and the cold colder.

6. Make the hot stage as hot as you can. Often, not using enough heat is the reason contrast therapy is less effective. If your heat source cools during the process, consider having a newly heated one on standby or have someone who can reheat it for you during the one-minute cold stage.

7. During the warm phase, move the joint or stretch the muscle if possible.

8. Start and end with the cold phase.

9. Hot and cold therapy should be done once or twice a day until the injury is healed.

10. If the therapy causes you pain or discomfort, perhaps your temperatures are too intense, or perhaps you will need a different method of treatment – listen to your body.

Prepare yourself that the pain of the injury will return several hours after treatment, especially in the early days after the injury. If there is no improvement after three days of contrast temperature therapy, you may need to see a doctor.

Do contrast showers work for treating injuries?

Contrast showers are great for general health and well-being but not as effective for treating an injury. For contrast therapy to be beneficial for injuries, there needs to be a greater intensity in the contrasting temperatures than can be achieved in a shower.

When is it not a good idea to use contrast temperature therapy to treat an injury?

- Acute injuries are best treated with cold exposure *only* for the first three days. After that, contrast therapy can be used.
- Don't use contrast therapy on an open wound or damaged skin, as it can increase the risk of bleeding and infection. This includes scrapes, cuts, burns, boils, cysts, carcinoma, and sunburn.
- If you suffer from poor circulation, low blood pressure, or have a heart condition, you may have a negative reaction to extreme cold or heat.
- If you suffer from cold urticaria, hives may form on your skin after exposure to cold therapy.
- If you have a fever or infection, heat application may exacerbate the symptoms.
- Diabetic neuropathy or peripheral neuropathy reduces the ability to feel pain, so you may not be aware that you are damaging your skin with ice or heat.
- If you have Raynaud's syndrome, cold

treatments would adversely affect you as the condition is characterized by constricted blood vessels in colder temperatures.

The medical conditions listed above serve as a guide. Consult your doctor to enquire whether hot and cold therapy is right for you and the injury you have sustained.

Once you have the all-clear from your doctor, the biggest risk around contrast temperature therapy is that of burns. Only use hot and cold temperatures that you can tolerate. Your skin may turn bright red due to the hot and cold temperatures; however, a dark red color indicates the skin is being burned.

WHAT ARE THE RISKS OF CONTRAST TEMPERATURE THERAPY?

The negative side effects of getting too hot for too long

Whether you are in a desert, tropical jungle, hot tub, or sauna, if you get too hot for too long, your body will experience some negative side effects.

Dehydration

Even if you are soaking in a hot tub full of water or sitting in a steamy sauna, you can become dehydrated if you don't drink enough water. Don't be fooled into thinking that your risk of dehydration is any less because you're moving between hot and cold exposure. The only way to combat dehydration is to drink water. Dehydration can occur if you have been in a hot environment for too long.

Symptoms of dehydration:

- Dry mouth
- Thirst
- Dark yellow urine
- Headache
- Muscle cramps
- Dizziness
- Rapid heartbeat
- Rapid breathing
- Lack of energy
- Sleepiness
- Fainting

Heat stress

Once again, heat stress can occur even if you are moving between a hot and cold environment, especially if your hot environment is too hot or you stay there too long. I'm specifically referring to extremely hot environments like baths, tubs, and saunas where your body is 'immersed' in the heat.

Symptoms of heat stress:

- Dizziness or fainting
- Fatigue
- Headache
- Nausea
- Excessive sweating (which will lead to dehydration)
- Muscle cramps
- Lack of alertness

Lowered blood pressure

We've learned that one of the body's responses to heat is dilated blood vessels. This is great when you're practicing contrast exposure, and the cold exposure causes your blood vessels to contract again, causing the pumping action that stimulates improved circulation. However, if your blood vessels remain dilated for too long, your blood pressure will drop.

Symptoms of low blood pressure:

- Dizziness or lightheadedness
- Nausea
- Blurred vision
- Fainting

Inasmuch as you should take care not to allow yourself to become overexposed to the cold, you need to be aware of the dangers of overexposure to heat. Do not participate in any practice that involves immersion in hot water or sitting in a sauna if you suffer from heart conditions, are taking medication, or have other adverse health conditions.

The negative side effects of getting too cold for too long

I have already elaborated on the dangers of cold exposure throughout the book. Still, in the context of contrast temperature therapy, I'd like to remind you of the very real danger of hypothermia. If you jump into a frozen lake or a tub filled with ice-cold water, regardless of whether you were in a hot tub or sauna first, you are at risk of hypothermia if you remain immersed in the icy water for too long.

The cold will kill you *quicker* than the heat can. Depending on how cold it is, hypothermia can set in in as little as five minutes. Hypothermia can affect your core body temperature and then your brain, which means if you stay in the water too long, your brain may eventually be unable to tell your body it's time to get out.

Never practice cold exposure on your own

If you choose to practice contrast temperature therapy, there are a few things to keep in mind:

- You don't need to own a sauna and live near an icy lake to take advantage of the health benefits that contrast temperature therapy offers. A shower that goes from hot to cold is sufficient. Full immersion is optimal but not essential.
- Whichever method you choose, finish off with cold exposure—that is the one that leaves you feeling energized and revitalized.
- Both extremes of hot and cold can be very dangerous.
- Don't practice extreme contrast temperature therapy on your own, especially not outdoors.
- If you have a heart condition, you're on medication, or you are pregnant, don't practice contrast temperature therapy.
- Speak to your doctor before you add contrast temperature therapy to your daily routine.

8

FREQUENTLY ASKED QUESTIONS

There are many frequently asked questions about cold exposure or cryotherapy. Here, I answer the most common questions to clear any doubts you may have about kick-starting your cold exposure routine.

What are the negative side effects of cold exposure?

Depending on what type of cold exposure you practice, there may be any number of negative side effects.

Localized ice treatment: Numbness, tingling, redness, and irritation of the skin. However, these side effects are almost always temporary. If any of these symptoms persist for longer than 24 hours, see a doctor.

Cryo machines: Apart from some numbness, tingling, redness, or skin irritation, the biggest danger of using cryotherapy machines would be asphyxiation if liquid nitrogen is used in a space that is not well ventilated.

Cold water shower: There are no negative side effects associated with taking a cold shower unless your immune system is already compromised, in which case you may become more ill than before you took a shower.

Ice-cold water immersion: The biggest and very real danger of ice-cold water immersion is *hypothermia*. Also associated with immersion in any body of water is the danger of drowning. Never practice cold water immersion in an open body of water by yourself.

Outdoor cold exposure: *Hypothermia* is a very real risk, as well as frostbite and chilblains.

Additional Cold Exposure side effects

1) Cold exposure burns calories and accelerates your metabolic rate, so it can make you very hungry.

It doesn't matter how much fat you burn if you make up for it by over-eating. Furthermore, if you overdo cold exposure or become stressed out, you risk reducing thyroid performance, thereby slowing down your metabolism.

2) Although the cold doesn't seem to suppress immunity straightaway, it might do so when merged with intense physical effort or over-exposure.

Intense exercise is known to decrease immune function momentarily. So, if you are sick, you could get sicker, more easily. The same applies to cold exposure.

3) Viruses are more widespread in colder conditions, which makes them survive for longer.

Human rhinoviruses, such as the common cold, reproduce at temperatures lower than 98.6°F (37°C). If you're continuously freezing or hypothyroid, your body may cool to such a degree that it makes it easier for viruses to survive.

Further, while cooling yourself down during a fever may lower your body temperature, it also reduces some of the healing procedures the increased temperature is trying to achieve.

4) Cold exposure may reduce testosterone levels in men.

Maintaining the testicular area between 88-99°F (31-37°C) improves sperm production and RNA, DNA, and protein synthesis.

5) Too much ice-cold exposure can cause neuropathy in your toes and fingers.

Neuropathy is weakness, numbness, and pain that is

caused by nerve damage—usually in the hands and feet. Urticaria, chilblains, and frostbite are similar negative outcomes of over-exposure to icy-cold conditions. Generally, a quick cold shower or even an ice bath for five to ten minutes won't cause these negative side effects. Usually, they occur as a result of persistent cold exposure, getting exposed to the cold while your immune system is weak, or other stressors.

Is it safe to practice cold exposure during pregnancy?

No, it is not.

According to a study by researchers at the National Institutes of Health, being exposed to extreme hot or cold temperatures during pregnancy may raise the risk of preterm birth[1].

The researchers discovered that women who underwent extreme cold exposure during the first seven weeks of their pregnancies had a 20% higher chance of delivering before 34 weeks of pregnancy, a 9% increased chance for delivering between 34-36 weeks, and a 3% increased chance for delivering in weeks 37 and 38.

This indicates that pregnant women should avoid exposure to extremely cold temperatures.

Can people with heart conditions practice cold exposure?

As with all medical conditions, and before you attempt any new healthcare routine, speak to your doctor first. If you have a heart condition, you may be able to benefit from cold exposure in the form of a contrast therapy shower, but you will probably not be able to participate in extreme cold immersion, and that includes cryotherapy chambers.

If you compare your blood to ketchup, exposure to cold temperatures causes ketchup to thicken. In the same way, prolonged or excessive cold exposure can cause your blood to thicken, raise blood pressure, reduce the flow of blood to the heart, and cause blood clots to form.

Hot showers versus cold showers: Which one is better?

If your body craves a hot shower in the morning, you're not alone. Most people crank the handle all the way up and relish standing under the hot water. Studies show that cold showers offer a variety of health benefits over hot showers, so I believe they should be part of your daily routine.

The following list details the benefits of cold and hot showers:

Cold Shower:

- Reduces skin damage from pollution, strengthens skin's natural barrier, and improves cell reproduction
- Boosts your immune system
- Closes pores and tightens skin
- Reduces hair loss
- Helps muscles recover after a workout
- Relieves itchy skin
- Aids in weight loss

Hot Shower:

- Relaxes muscles and eases joint pain
- Clears nasal passage

- Reduces inflammation and puffiness
- Helps you sleep better
- Opens pores leading to cleaner skin
- Relieves headaches and has a calming effect
- Reduces tiredness and fatigue

Are there any contraindications to cryotherapy?

You are advised **not to undergo** whole-body cryotherapy if you have any of the following conditions:

1. Arrhythmia
2. Acute or recent myocardial infarction
3. Symptomatic cardiovascular disease
4. Peripheral arterial occlusive disease
5. Cold allergies
6. Unstable angina pectoris
7. Severe hypertension (blood pressure over 180/100)
8. Venous thrombosis
9. Raynaud's disease
10. Acute or recent cerebrovascular accident
11. Uncontrolled seizures
12. Fever
13. Tumor(s)

14. Symptomatic lung disorders
15. Severe anemia
16. Infection
17. Bleeding disorders
18. Severe claustrophobia
19. Acute kidney and urinary tract diseases

Parental permission is required for anyone 18 years or younger. Also, it is important to avoid whole-body cryotherapy if you are pregnant or have a pacemaker fitted.

Are there risks associated with cryotherapy?

Yes, there are.

Tissue damage, ranging from mild to frostbite, can occur. Research states that frostbite can be severe in people with conditions that reduce sensitivity to feelings and sensations, for example, people with diabetes or any conditions that affect their nerves[2]. They may be unable to fully feel its effect, which could lead to further nerve damage.

People with severe heart conditions may also be at risk[3].

The most common side effects are redness or skin irritation, an allergic reaction to the cold, frostbite, or skin burns.

According to the Washington Post[4], 26 October 2015, a salon worker entered a cryotherapy chamber alone and unattended and was found dead inside ten hours later. While her passing is tragic, medical experts could not determine what caused her death since she was alone.

As with any health or fitness product or medical procedure, discretion and discernment are advised. Before trying cryotherapy, visit your doctor to determine if you have any health conditions that preclude you from participating in this type of activity.

What does frostbite look like, and how is it treated?

Frostbitten skin is numb and cold and can appear white, bluish-white, red, grayish-yellow, brown, purple, or black, depending on how severe the frostbite is. If left untreated, frostbite will turn to gangrene. Treatment may include the following: rewarming the skin in warm water, oral pain medicine, oral antibiotics to prevent infection, and whirlpool therapy to speed up healing. In extreme cases where tissue damage is severe, the damaged tissue must be surgically removed, or worse still, the damaged body part must be amputated.

During rewarming, users may experience burning, swelling, and stinging. In cases of more serious frost-bite, fluid-filled blisters may emerge hours to days after rewarming.

Can I do cryotherapy if I am claustrophobic?

Yes, you can, especially if you opt for a cryotherapy chamber that doesn't enclose your head. Some cryotherapy machines are like a small, enclosed room— that won't work if you're claustrophobic. Be sure to enquire what type of machine is used before you make an appointment for treatment.

A cryotherapy technician will be on hand to assist you while you are in the chamber, and, should you wish to get out, you can simply and easily push the door open.

Do I need to work out before cold exposure?

No, you don't. Although cryotherapy is a popular workout recovery therapy practiced by athletes, you don't need to get all hot and sweaty beforehand to benefit from cryotherapy. Ultimately, it's your choice. The ideal time for cold exposure is when it's most beneficial for you.

While on the subject of cold exposure and exercise, I would *not* recommend exercising after cold exposure. You can strain, pull or tear a muscle if you force it into a stretch while it is cold.

I've heard people use cryotherapy for anti-aging – is it true?

Yes! Many people, including A-list celebrities undergo cryotherapy as part of their anti-aging routine. It helps with cellular regeneration, circulation, and collagen production.

When you have finished a cryo-sauna treatment, newly-oxygenated blood moves through your body, which helps it produce collagen. Collagen is a protein that is found in bones, muscles, skin, and tendons. It's what makes our skin glow. It also helps to keep the skin strong and helps to regenerate new skin cells.

As we age, our collagen production drops. Toxins, like smoking, and exposure to the sun reduce collagen levels.

What should I use if I don't have a plunge pool?

You can use any large tub, provided it's big enough for you to get neck-deep under ice water—even if it means you have to crouch or lie down. Although being comfortable is important, you won't be in the tub for more than a few minutes at a time, so your seating or standing position is not as important as how much of your body can be immersed. I know someone who uses a cattle feeder trough. I also have a friend who uses a wheelie bin and another who uses a kiddie's pool. You could use a chest freezer too. After all, where there's a will, there's a way.

Things to consider if you use a chest freezer:

- You can set the thermostat so that the water stays at a constant 50°F (10°C)—this is the temperature at which the benefits of cold-water exposure begin.
- On days that you want to do a shorter-colder exposure, you can turn the thermostat down to cool the water a few hours before you take the plunge.
- On the downside, you need electricity to keep the water temperature constant, which will push up your utility bill.
- **Always unplug the freezer** before you get in.

- **Never close the lid** while you are in the freezer.

My heart rate is unsteady. Can I still take cold-water swims?

"I had my mitral valve repaired a few years ago, and my heart rate is sometimes unsteady. Can I still swim in cold water?"

The shock of cold water against the skin activates a fight-or-flight response. The adrenal glands pump out extra adrenaline (epinephrine) and other stress hormones. They cause blood vessels to narrow. This preserves heat, but it moves even more blood to the chest, placing strain on the heart. Extra epinephrine also tends to interrupt the heart's steady rhythm.

Generally speaking, this isn't a problem in someone with a healthy heart, but it could create trouble for someone who is susceptible to arrhythmias. In addition, the colder the water, the higher the diving response. This leads to a lower heart rate and higher blood pressure.

Know your limits, and don't take any undue risks. Seek medical advice before you try cold water emersion. Always submerge in the presence of someone who can pull you to safety and knows how to do CPR. Be on the lookout for symptoms of a slow heart rate or an arrhythmia, such as feeling faint or noticing unsteady or "missed" heartbeats. If you observe these symptoms, immediately exit the water and seek medical attention.

My skin is allergic to cold temperatures. Should I practice cold exposure?

Have you ever experienced an itchy rash or felt faint after being in cold water? Do you grow welts on your skin from the cold? If you answered yes to either of these questions, you might have a medical condition known as cold urticaria. People who have this medical condition grow welts (hives on their skin that generally itch) when exposed to the cold. If you've had a negative reaction to cold temperatures, such as feeling faint or having difficulty breathing, it's important to find out if you have cold urticaria. If you have these types of allergic reactions, ask your doctor or general physician for advice.

I have severe migraine attacks. Should I take cold showers?

If your body is sensitive to cold water and you suffer from migraines, consult your physiotherapist or doctor before taking cold showers. Many people who have migraines are sensitive to the cold. Participating in cold therapy or taking a cold shower can cause a migraine. When you have a migraine, keep away from cold showers, as they can make you feel fatigued and increase your pain.

Follow the steps listed below if you want to take a cold shower, but only after your doctor's consent:

1. Start with lukewarm water (or slightly colder), as you must be gentle. If the water is too cold, your muscles will tense, potentially increasing your migraine.
2. Try a navy shower. Turn the tap off after you are wet, apply soap, then turn the tap back on to rinse off. This isn't advisable in winter, but it works well in summer.
3. A short cool rinse at the end of your shower can help revitalize you. Just avoid being so cold that your muscles tense.

I suffer from stress and anxiety. Should I take cold showers?

Anxiety is a mental health condition that causes worries and fears. While some anxiety and stress are a normal part of life, anxiety disorders can hinder a person's daily activities, sometimes making it harder for them to participate in work and social activities.

Cold showers help to enhance blood circulation. When you cool your body temperature, your body responds by circulating fresh blood. Anxiety may cause a rise in blood pressure. So, in theory, a cold shower may help to bring your blood pressure down.

Another way cold showers may help with stress and anxiety is by activating endorphins, which are also known as the 'feel-good' hormones in your brain. Endorphins can alleviate symptoms of anxiety and depression. Cold water may also lessen cortisol, a stress-inducing hormone.

Athletes use extreme cold showers to help reduce the inflammation that may lead to muscle spasms after an intense workout. For anxiety, a cold shower may lead to similar benefits in terms of inflammation. Ongoing stress may raise inflammation, which can then lead to a round of inflammation-induced anxiety.

Also, a cold shower can momentarily take your mind off the things you are fearful or worried about. For example, the minutes you devote to thinking about how the cold water feels on your body may act as a mindfulness practice, grounding you in the moment as opposed to focusing on future or past events that are out of your control.

When using cold showers for anxiety, you should only do so for a few minutes at a time. You can then end your shower with lukewarm water.

I suffer from depression. Can cold therapy help?

In short, yes!

Whole-body cryotherapy results in the release of hormones, including adrenaline and endorphins[5] (the 'feel-good' hormones in your brain). So, this treatment has a positive effect on depression. At least one study has proven the effectiveness of whole-body cryotherapy as a short-term treatment for depression[6].

Will a cold shower before bedtime help me sleep?

In short, not really.

Our bodies are managed by a 24-hour master clock called a circadian rhythm. This body clock informs us when it's time for bed, time to wake, and even when to eat. It's accountable for bodily functions, hormone levels, and more. At night, the clock sends messages to our bodies that it's time for bed. One way it does this is by reducing our core temperature by about one degree.

So, how does this relate to showering? If you take a warm shower, your body will cool down as soon as you leave the water and dry off. Unless your shower was too hot—then you will need between 45minutes to an hour to cool down properly before you can sleep.

Now, you may be thinking that a cold shower will speed up the process of cooling down, and this is true up to a point. But remember, cold showers and ice baths have an energizing effect, so rather save them for the morning hours or, at the latest, early in the afternoon.

Does cold exposure cause damage to my testicles?

We're aware that male genitals respond to cold conditions by shrinking. But honestly, your private parts prefer cooler temperatures. In fact, sperm production is most optimal when testes are a few degrees cooler than your core temperature—that's probably why they hang down a little, away from the body. When your testicles get too hot, the quality of your sperm can be harmed.

This being said, they can get *too cold*, which also has a negative impact on the health of your sperm[7].

Not only for the sake of your testicles but for every other extremity, treat the cold with respect and practice extreme cold exposure with caution.

Are cold showers beneficial for fibromyalgia?

The Wim Hof Method[8] has been found to offer relief from the symptoms of fibromyalgia. One of the instructors, Tom Stijven, suffered from fibromyalgia and found relief in the Wim Hof Method, which includes a combination of cold exposure, proper breathing, and commitment.

Another supporter of cold shower relief for fibromyalgia is The Fibro Guy[9]. He states, "What I find most beneficial for people with Fibromyalgia is that… a cold shower can give a good 90 minutes of total pain relief in most people. This gives you an opportunity to have… a 'normal' morning…."

Don't let excuses stop you from living a healthier, more vital life.

Cold exposure is going mainstream and is even carving a niche in the fitness travel industry. In recent years, many countries, including Norway, Sweden, and Denmark, whose inhabitants have skinny-dipped in cold lakes under the midnight sun for generations, have become popular destinations for those embarking on a full-body health and wellness expedition that comprises cold exposure.

LEAVE A 1-CLICK REVIEW

I would be incredibly grateful if you could take just 60 seconds to write a brief review on Amazon, even if it's just a few sentences

Scan the QR code to leave a quick review:

AFTERWORD

"Consistency is the secret to results that last."

An ancient Greek parable famously known as the Sorites Paradox talks about the results one small step can have when replicated enough times.

One version of the paradox goes as follows: Can one coin make a person wealthy? If you offer a person a pile of ten coins, would you say that they are rich? But what if you add another coin? And another? And another? Eventually, you will have to acknowledge that the addition of a coin made the person rich.

We can say the same about healthy habits like cold exposure. Can one tiny change revolutionize your life? It's unlikely. But what if you made another? And another? And another? Eventually, you will have to acknowledge that your life was transformed by one small change. People have used cold water therapies for centuries as a treatment to revitalize and improve their overall wellbeing. In Chapters 1 and 2, I mentioned some scientific studies that support the beneficial effects of cold showers on mental and physical health.

Throughout the book, we looked at scientific evidence in support of cold exposure. We learned about the increasing popularity of cold exposure and how its benefits are not reserved for professional athletes, business moguls, and A-list celebrities.

Unfortunately, most people are stuck in the *'no change'* equation:

comfortable = complacent = no change

This is not an ideal way to live, and you will not be able to live life to the full if you stay there. I aim to improve in all aspects of my life steadily. I am happiest when I am progressing.

If you want to do something meaningful and fulfilling in life, like starting your own business or learning a new skill, you will probably face some difficult times. It's a mistake to assume that following your passion will always be easy. We must push through difficult times, and sometimes we must do things we don't want to do —that's when we grow.

Success is not a target that can be reached or a finish line that can be crossed. It requires ongoing development and enhancement; it is a continuous process of refinement.

Remember what I mentioned in Chapter 6: if you're having difficulty changing your habits, the cause isn't you – it's your system. Bad habits replicate again and again, not because you don't want to change, but because you have the wrong system for change.

Understanding the Habit Loop – cue, craving, response, and reward – will help you construct better systems and develop better habits.

- At first, you may not even want to start cold exposure in a bid to postpone the commitment – you must push through and make it work.
- Sometimes it will be tough to stick to the habit once you have begun – you'll have to find a way to make it interesting.
- Other times you won't feel like continuing – you'll need to find ways to make it rewarding.

Life enrichment is an ongoing process. Whenever you're looking for motivation to continue, refer to the Habit Loop to keep yourself going. Make it enjoyable. Make it worthwhile. Always look for the next way to get 1% better.

The secret to getting results that last forever is to never stop making adjustments. It's amazing what you can achieve if you don't quit. Remember, even tiny habits compound and lead to extraordinary results.

The mind is a battlefield. The first step to attaining success in any endeavor is getting your head in the game. Without the right mindset, well-thought-out plans can fail; with the right mindset, nothing is impossible.

Many people try and fail and then try again to introduce new health and wellness habits into their daily routine. Some succeed. What is the difference between those who try and fail and quit?—And those who try and fail and try again until they eventually succeed?

Those who succeed make up their minds to do so!

Do you dream of a better life and long to feel healthier and have more vitality?

Dreaming and longing, or thinking and wishing, don't result in the realization of goals. However, if you can adjust your thinking, you can turn your thoughts and ideas into plans and goals that will result in lasting success.

That's the power of cold exposure—start small, stick to it, achieve big.

Be responsible when practicing cold exposure. The cold is a thrilling place that can bring much rejuvenation and healing, but if not treated with respect, it can hurt you, make you ill, or kill you.

Cold exposure is not intended to be a macho thing where you get to prove how brave and resilient you are. When practiced regularly and correctly, it is a healthy lifestyle-improving modality, a character builder, a personal-goal enhancer.

Respect the cold! Love the cold! Utilize the cold!

Now you understand how cryotherapy works and how it can benefit you, give it a go. If you benefited from this book, please leave a review and tell other people about it.

I wish you the very best of luck in your cold therapy journey.

James H. Smart

JUST FOR YOU...

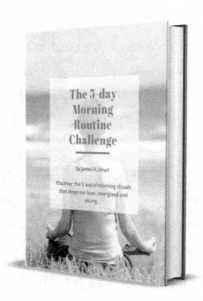

A FREE GIFT FOR OUR READERS

The 5-Day Morning Routine Challenge.
Discover the 5 weird morning rituals that keep me lean,
energized and young.
Start today by visiting the link:
www.jameshsmart.com

RESOURCES

1. THE SCIENCE OF COLD EXPOSURE

1. Patrick, R.P., Ph.D. Cold exposure Blog. Available from: https://www.foundmyfitness.com/topics/cold-exposure-therapy
2. Lademann, H. PDF Available from https://www.mdpi.com › pdf 4 August 2021
3. Ferrucci, L., Fabbri, E. Inflammageing: chronic inflammation in ageing, cardiovascular disease, and frailty. Nat Rev Cardiol 15, 505–522 (2018). https://doi.org/10.1038/s41569-018-0064-2
4. Hirvonen, H.E., Mikkelsson, M.K., Kautiainen, H., Pohjolainen, T.H., Leirisalo-Repo, M. National Library of Medicine. May/June 2006. Article available from: https://pubmed.ncbi.nlm.nih.gov/16870097/
5. Nurs, J.N. National Library of Medicine. 10 October 2017. Article available from: https://pubmed.ncbi.nlm.nih.gov/28880416/
6. Garcia, C., Karri, J., Nicholas, A.Z., Adb-Elsayed, A. Use of Cryotherapy for Managing Chronic Pain: An Evidence-Based Narrative. 14 December 2020. Available from: https://link.springer.com/article/10.1007/s40122-020-00225-w

2. THE PHYSICAL AND MENTAL BENEFITS OF COLD EXPOSURE

1. Greenhill, C. 6 August 2013. Obesity: Cold exposure increases brown adipose tissue in humans. https://pubmed.ncbi.nlm.nih.gov/23917582/
2. van Marken Lichtenbelt, W. 17 October 2011. Human Brown Fat Obesity. https://www.ncbi.nlm.nih.gov/pmc/articles/PMC3356108/

3. Wilderness & Environmental Medicine, ISSN: 1080-6032, Vol: 22, Issue: 4, Page: 343-351
   Publication Year 2011
4. Shevchuk NA, Radoja S. Possible stimulation of anti-tumor immunity using repeated cold stress: a hypothesis. Infect Agent Cancer. 2007;2:20. Published 2007 Nov 13. doi:10.1186/1750-9378-2-20
5. Rowlatt J. 19 October 2020. Could cild water hold a clue to a dementia cure? https://www.bbc.com/news/health-54531075
6. Liu, Y., Hu, W., Murakawa, Y. Cold-induced RNA-binding proteins regulate circadian gene expression by controlling alternative polyadenylation. Sci Rep 3, 2054 (2013). https://doi.org/10.1038/srep02054
7. https://www.cancer.gov/about-cancer/treatment/types/surgery/cryosurgery

3. A COLD SHOWER A DAY KEEPS THE DOCTOR AWAY

1. Shevchuk, N.A. Adapted cold shower as a potential treatment for depression. Med Hypotheses. 2008. https://www.sciencedirect.com/science/article/abs/pii/S030698770700566X
2. Machado A.F., Ferreira P.H., Micheletti J.K., de Almeida A.C., Lemes I.R., Vanderlei F.M., Netto J. Junior & Pastre C.M. 18 November 2015. https://link.springer.com/article/10.1007/s40279-015-0431-7

4. TAKE IT TO THE NEXT LEVEL

1. Lombardi, G., Ziemann, E., and Banfil, G. 2 May 2017. Whole-Body Cryotherapy in Athletes. https://www.ncbi.nlm.nih.gov/pmc/articles/PMC5411446/
2. Polaris Market Research May 2020. https://www.polarismarketresearch.com/industry-analysis/cryotherapy-market

18 The Reduction of Distress Using Therapeutic Geothermal Water Procedures in a Randomized Controlled Clinical Trial - Scientific Figure on ResearchGate. Available from: https://www.researchgate.net/figure/Human-response-to-stress-curve-according-to-Nixon-P-Practitioner-1979-Yerkes-RM_fig2_274901016

5. GET COMFORTABLE BEING UNCOMFORTABLE

1.
2. https://www.ted.com/talks/kelly_mcgonigal_how_to_-make_stress_your_friend/up-next?language=en
3. Schwabe, L., and Schächinger, H. 10 March 2018. National Library of Medicine. https://pubmed.ncbi.nlm.nih.gov/29573884/
4. Minkley N., Schrödera1 T.P., Wolf O.T., Kirchnera W.H., 22 March 2014. Science Direct. https://www.sciencedirect.com/science/article/abs/pii/S0306453014001188#!

6. FORMING A NEW HABIT

1. Leaf Dr. C., 3 October 2018. https://drleaf.com/blogs/news/you-are-not-a-victim-of-your-biology
2. McLeod, S.A.14 January 2018. Edward Thorndike. Simply Psychology. https://www.simplypsychology.org/edward-thorndike.html
3. Charles Duhigg and Nir Eyal deserve special recognition for their influence on this image. This representation of the habit loop is a combination of language that was popularized by Duhigg's book, The Power of Habit, and a design that was popularized by Eyal's book, Hooked.

7. CONTRAST TEMPERATURE THERAPY

1. Sears, B. 22 June 2020. Whirlpool use in Physical Therapy. https://www.verywellhealth.com/whirlpool-use-in-physical-therapy-2696642

2. Feloni, R. 25 October 2017. https://www.businessinsider.com/tony-robbins-daily-sauna-cold-plunge-combo-benefits-2017-10?IR=T

3. Martins, A. 12 January 2021. Why you should take contrasting showers. https://asweatlife.com/2021/01/contrasting-showers/

8. FREQUENTLY ASKED QUESTIONS

1. Ha, Sandie & Liu, Danping & Zhu, Yeyi & Kim, Sung & Sherman, Seth & Mendola, Pauline. 2016. Ambient Temperature and Early Delivery of Singleton Pregnancies. Environmental Health Perspectives. 125. 10.1289/EHP97.

2. Gotter A. The benefits of Cryotherapy. 2 March 2020. https://www.healthline.com/health/cryotherapy-benefits#benefits

3. PureAire Monitoring Systems. 14 December 2015 https://www.pureairemonitoring.com/the-hidden-dangers-and-facts-of-cryotherapy-how-to-remain-safe-and-get-health-benefits-too/

4. https://www.washingtonpost.com/news/morning-mix/wp/2015/10/26/salon-worker-praised-cryotherapy-then-froze-to-death-during-treatment/

5. Gotter A. The benefits of Cryotherapy. 2 March 2020. https://www.healthline.com/health/cryotherapy-benefits#benefits

6. Shevchuk NA. Adapted cold shower as a potential treatment for depression. Med Hypotheses. 2008. https://www.ncbi.nlm.nih.gov/pmc/articles/PMC2734249/

7. Roland J. 2 January 2020. Why Are My Testicles Cold and What's the Best Way to Warm Them Up? https://www.healthline.com/health/cold-testicles-2#optimal-temp

8. https://www.wimhofmethod.com/fibromyalgia-relief
9. https://www.thefibroguy.com/blog/are-cold-showers-good-for-fibromyalgia/